CANCER AND MENTAL ILLNESS

A Decade of Published Research
In Review (2014-2023)

By John H. Morgan

In memory of the late
Professor Angus Hawkins, Ph.D.,
Fellow of Keble College/Oxford.
My friend and colleague for 20 years
at Oxford University.

CANCER AND MENTAL ILLNESS

A Decade of Published Research In Review (2014-2023)

By John H. Morgan
Ph.D. (Hartford), D.Sc. (London), Psy.D.(FH/Oxford)
Senior Fellow in Behavioral Science (*emeritus*)
Foundation House/Oxford (UK)
Professor of Clinical Psychopathology *(retired)*

ISBN 978-155605-546-1 Paperback

ISBN 978-155605-547-8 E Book

Table of Contents

INTRODUCTION

Mental Illness and Psychiatric Disorders

A Convergent Analysis in Cancer Research

The challenge for psychiatric oncology in diagnosing and treating a cancer patient suffering from mental illness constitutes an enduring opportunity to confront the mind-body conundrum. What is happening to the cancerous body which is concomitantly affecting and being affected by the mental state of the patient is the matrix of research addressed in this critical review of published scholarship. All cancer patients do not suffer from mental health issues nor do all patients suffering from mental illness have cancer. However, the fact that upwards of 35% of all cancer patients suffer from some manifestation of mental illness according to the National Cancer Institute lends urgency to a robust study of the connection between cancer and mental illness. The spectrum of mental health issues range from mild mental disorders such as anxiety and depression to severe mental illnesses such as schizophrenia and debilitating paranoia. Though interest in this subject reaches back to the 1950s this present review of scholarship will focus on the most recently published research in the medical journals since 2014.

In this study we will explore the meaning and significance of the distinctive use of "mental illness" and "psychiatric disorders" as diagnostic classifications relevant to the linkage of cancer to the patient's mental state. It is generally understood that this distinction of illness rather than disorder is more readily utilized by oncologists for "medical" conditions than by psychologists for "behavioral" issues. A question to be examined is to what extent, if any, there is an emphasis upon the "medical" nature of the classification of mental illness versus the "psychotherapeutic" emphasis on mental disorders, the former being clearly characterized as a "medical" classification whereas the latter is more clearly designated a "behavioral" classification.

A simple attempt at determining the preferred term within the medical and psychiatric communities was made by identify the frequency of use of "mental illness" and "mental disorders" in the major repositories of published scholarship within these professions. We found that "mental ill" was more commonly employed in PubMed and that "mental disorder" was dominant in PubPsych. Though not officially determinative, nevertheless, the preference for one term over another is clearly linked to the type of professional practice engaged in the use of these two terms. One looming sidebar in this attempt to differentiate the labeling process is the place of the cost of healthcare coverage as that coverage might be linked to the label employed in the treatment protocol. Owing to the absence of any scientifically acceptable evidentiary validation of the linkage between the biochemistry of cancer and the psychopathology of mental illness, the profoundly massive and expansive presence of the psychosocial spectrum of cancer care constitutes the basis upon which continued serious research is occurring. It might just be that psychiatric oncology could serve as a mediator between the medical designation on the one hand and the psychotherapeutic designation on the other.

One subtle ambiguity in nomenclature in the area of diagnostic designations has to do with the mixed and confused frequently interchangeable use of the terms "severe" and "serious" when applied to mental illness and mental disorders. The most common trend is to identify anxiety and depression as a form of mild mental illness where as such mental disorders as bipolar, schizophrenia, and clinically diagnosed psychotic disorders are commonly labeled severe mental illness (SMI). A further refinement has recently emerged in which severe psychiatric illness (SPI) includes generally schizophrenia, schizoaffective and psychotic disorders, bipolar disorders and even major depressive disorders. What will become increasingly clear and baffling through this investigation is the interchangeability of the diagnostic classifications of "mental illness" and "mental disorder." In this opening essay, it is our intention to deepened and broaden these distinctions without making a claim to have solved the issue, but only making it more interesting. The greatest challenge initially will be to navigate between the competing perspectives of the medical community (AMA) and the psychotherapeutic community (APA) in classifying this broad behavioral matrix as either a mental "illness" or a mental "disorder." Short of resolving the issue, we will at least attempt to make the rationale for the distinctions clear from both the medical and psychological perspectives.

As will be seen in the following detailed critical review of key research articles dealing with the relationship between cancer and the behavioral well-being of the patient, it is clearly obvious that there is no clinical evidence of a biochemical linkage between cancer and the mental state of the patient such that the psychosocial characteristics of the patient constitute the basis for a causal linkage. Because 35% of all Americans suffer from some form of mental disorder (according to the APA) and 35% of all cancer patients suffer from some sort of mental illness (according to the NCI), it is a common suggestion that there is clearly a correlational link between these two statistical realities. The most generally recognized authority regarding the definitional issues related to mental illness and mental disorders is that of Stedman, Thomas Lathrop Stedman's (2005, 2nd ed.), *The American Heritage Stedman's Medical Dictionary.* Stedman puts forth extreme effort to offer a distinctive clarification of the meaning and differences between mental disorders and mental illness, an effort enthusiastically applauded though offering little real resolution to the professional disputes involved. "Mental disorders" as a labeling classification, according to Stedman, is essentially outdated due to its origins as a viable term in the early days of emerging psychiatry and psychiatric oncology. In a post-Kraepelinian world of modern medicine, we now understand that there is a matrix of confluent factors affecting the mind and the body as well as brain function such that the use of the concept of mental illness is fundamentally applied to an individual's overall mental wellbeing. However, on the other hand, the classificatory term commonly used today in psychiatric oncology is "mental illness" and is applied to a full spectrum of health issues affecting an individual's moods, cognitive processes, and behavior.

The prevalence of mental illness with psychiatric disorders among cancer patients is extremely high reaching upwards of 35% (Caruso, et al., 2017). The presence of mental illness within cancer patients who have had a history of psychiatric issues often constitutes a furthering of symptoms whereas patients without a history of emotional issues the diagnosis of cancer too often precipitates the emergence of latent psychiatric conditions which otherwise have remained dormant in the patient's life. The range of emotional responses to a cancer diagnosis spans the modest response of sadness and

worry to extreme manifestations of anxiety, depression, and post-traumatic stress disorders. A troubling scenario regarding the diagnosis of cancer and the emergence of mental illness and psychiatric issues is exacerbated by the failure of the oncology assessment and treatment team to recognize or discount mental health symptoms as a merely normal emotional response to the diagnostic experience (Grassi, Spiegel, Riba, 2017). Mental health issues too often have been responsible for cancer patients not complying with treatment directives owing to the overwhelming encounter with hopelessness, anxiety, and depression. Forsythe, Kent, Weaver, et al. (2013) have shown documentation demonstrating the negative results of a cancer diagnosis for a patient suffering from mental illness and, as Morgan has shown in his extensive study of the relationship between cancer and suicide (Morgan, 2023), the need for a greater emphasis upon recognition and development of responsive treatment protocols is called for within the oncology medical community. In the consistent absence of any verifiable biochemical linkage between cancer and mental illness, psychiatric oncologists have demonstrated repeatedly the psychosocial linkage between cancer and mental illness such that any ideological differences between the medical and psychotherapeutic terminology of mental illness and mental disorder seems more or less inconsequential in terms of determining a diagnosis and treatment protocol.

Many world health organizations have ventured into the troubled waters of definitional parameters of mental health dysfunctions, i.e., illness and/or disorder, and one of the more commonly referenced definitions has been provided by the National Institutes of Health (NIH) which defines a mental disorder as "a disturbance of normal functioning of the mind or body." Such disorders, according to the NIH, may trace their etiology to genetic factors, disease, or trauma. Recognizing that such disorders may have a negative impact upon not only the mind and body but upon the physical brain itself, the term "mental disorder" has become somewhat outdated and suspect in terms of its descriptive qualities. On the other hand, the medical community has gradually moved towards the utilization of the term "mental illness" which is more suggestive of the psychiatric conditions affecting not just the mind but the body and brain as well. A passing argument of slight dubious merit is that the term "disorder" too commonly implies a negative quality where as "illness" suggests a medical condition subject to treatment protocols. Since mental disorders are not simply etiologically linked to the psychosocial and physical environment of the patient, the American Psychiatric Association's *Diagnostic and Statistical Manual of Mental Disorders* (see DSM–IV–TR; DSM–5) and the World Health Organization's *International Classification of Diseases* have listed a roster of possible causes linked to physiological, genetic, chemical, social, and other factors. Still, the cognitive divide between the psychiatric community and the medical community continues to lead the latter to employ "illness" whereas the former clings to "disorder" as more relevant to their treatment protocols.

It is the Centers for Disease Control (CDC) that has moved the conversation to a more practical and pragmatic level of utilization by defining mental illness as a "condition that affects a person's think, feeling, mood, and behavior." The rationale for the use of "mental illness" rather than "mental disorders" as explained by the CDC is that the term "mental illness" implies in its use that mental health issues actually affect more than just the cognitive mental processes suggested in the term "mental disorder" such that mental health issues such as depression, anxiety, schizophrenia, and cognates of these are covered by the mental illness terminology. Granted that traditionalist physicians often still employ the terms of mental disorder and mental illness as synonyms, the most informed within the psychiatric profession are insistent upon the preference for the term mental illness. Relevant to the ascendency of the designation mental illness over mental disorder, the American Psychiatric Association's internationally distinguished resource compendium, i.e., DSM-V (Diagnostic and Statistical Manual of Mental Disorders-Revised Fifth Edition), has identified 357 types of mental illnesses which are diagnosable and this reference text DSM-V has risen to be the primary resource for consultancies in the U.S. for diagnostics (McNally, 2011).

CHAPTER ONE

Overview of the Mental Illness and Cancer Crisis

A major issue in cancer care throughout the world is the appalling disparity between the quality of care for lung cancer patients based on age and mental illness as key variables in treatment protocols, i.e., the older the patient and whether or not the patient has a mental disorder, constitutes the matrix of quality care. At one level the issue of cancer and mental illness forms a common linkage but another more exacerbating level has to do with the age of the cancer patient linked to a psychiatric disorder. Cara Bergamo of the Robert Wood Johnson Medical School in Camden, New Jersey, has been joined by oncology colleagues to specifically address what they have characterized as "inequalities" in the care of elderly lung cancer patients suffering from schizophrenia (Bergamo, Sigel, Mhango, Kale, Wisnivesky, 2014). Possibly owing to an inequality in assessment, diagnosis, and treatment protocols, the fact is statistically verified that cancer mortality is higher among individuals suffering from schizophrenia and to explore this reality more closely Bergamo and colleagues investigated the identifiable gaps in the diagnosis, treatment, and survival rate among lung cancer patients and particularly among elderly patients suffering from schizophrenia.

Relying upon a database of 96,702 patients with non-small cell lung cancer provided by the Surveillance, Epidemiology, and End Results databank (SEER) linked to records provided by Medicare for all patients being studied 66 years of age and older suffering from primary non-small cell lung cancer. Survival rates were compared using Kaplan-Meier methods to provide a comprehensively balanced study of this database. Studying both patients with and without schizophrenia, the team used unadjusted and multiple regression analyses drawing upon three categories, viz., lung cancer stage, diagnostic evaluation, and rates of stage-appropriate treatment.

Of the full database of 96,702 patients, 1.3% (n=1,303) had been diagnosed with schizophrenia and, compared to the general population, this grouping of elderly schizophrenic cancer patients manifested less late-stage disease when controlling for age, sex, marital status, race/ethnicity, income, histology, and comorbidities. These aging schizophrenic cancer patients were also less inclined to undergo appropriate evaluative assessments. Though the data showed that this particular grouping of cancer patients saw a decrease in survival rate there was no recorded difference when controlling for treatment. This research team found that the overall outcome for this grouping of elderly cancer patients with schizophrenia was linked to a reluctance on the part of the patient to access diagnostic evaluation resulting in delayed and minimalized treatment. The team was consistent in reminding researchers as well as practitioners that the range of treatment modalities in attending the needs of the geriatric schizophrenic cancer patient constitutes one of the monumental challenges to the care and treatment of these patients such that it commonly occurs that both treatment and assessment suffer in thoroughness thus exacerbating the overall health of the patient.

Discussed extensively in the introductory essay to this study is the linkage between mental disorders and cancer in which attention was given specifically to issues related to both mental disorders and mental illness. In the essay by O'Neill and colleagues at the University of Ulster (O'Neill, Posada-Villa, Medina-Mora, et al., 2014), his team probed the baffling question as to whether or not there is any identifiable linkage between life stages and gender of the cancer patient and, if so, what are the characteristics of such a linkage. Based on data provided by the World Mental Health Survey Initiative, O'Neill and colleagues assessed the prevalence of mental disorders in a face-to-face household population covering nineteen countries and including 52,095 respondents. Relying on self-reported diagnoses, these oncologists focused their attention on smoking and the overall history of tobacco use among the respondents. Of major significance in this data-based study was the identification of the onset of mental disorders among the survivors over time.

Comorbidity concerns constituted an overarching point of awareness as the research team was fully cognizant of the fact that poor mental health often impacts treatment protocols and successes particularly as postsurgical complications compare in frequency with survival-related outcomes impacting physical health as well as mental health. In their conclusions, the team called for a more careful consideration of the potential benefits of cognitive behavioral therapy as well as pharmacotherapy in the desire to optimize treatment efficacies as this particular study was able to effectively demonstrate that there is a linkage of relevance between mental health and bladder cancer which is worthy of noting and responding to with further research endeavors.

The driving research interest focused upon the nature and scope of the relationship between cancer and mental illness and the team was able to determine that adjusting for comorbidity in self-reporting respondents, panic disorders, particularly phobias, and alcohol abusive behavior were effectively linked to self-reported diagnosis of cancer such that the ratio of mental disorder respondents to those reporting a cancer diagnosis illustrated the onset of mental disorders following the initial diagnosis. This study dispelled the suspicion of a relationship between a specific cancer to a specific mental disorder preferring to argue that the relationship between cancer and mental disorders is of a generalized nature. They did discover that depression is reported earlier in a patient's life and more commonly among women including the presence of PTSD in early diagnosed patients.

This data-based study constitutes an early illustration of the dynamic relationship between mental disorders and self-reporting cancer diagnoses in which such relevant information as the presence of comorbidity, gender, and stages of life issues are embraced in the analysis. Early identification of mental disorders among diagnosed cancer patients is emphasized in these findings.

One of the major research challenges and interests in this matrix of cancer and mental health has to do with the comparison of patients diagnosed with cancer who were suffering from a mental health issue and those who were not at the time of diagnosis. Always of relevance is the stage of cancer at the time of diagnosis and the comorbidity of the patient in terms of mental health issues. Chin-Kuo Change of King's College London's Institute of Psychiatry was joined with several of his colleagues precisely to investigate this matrix of converging issues (Chang, Hayes, et al., 2014). Of particular interest to this team of oncologists was the relationship between the state of cancer diagnosis and the rate of survival when linked to mental illness of the cancer patient. Accessing a London database of 28,477 cancer patients over the age of 15 with identified cancer, the team found 2,206 patients had been previously assessed and treated for secondary mental healthcare issues prior to their cancer diagnosis of which 125 were treated for severe mental illnesses including schizophrenia, schizoaffective or bipolar disorders.

In an attempt to determine whether or not and, if so, to what extent there exists a corroborating correlation between cancer patients diagnosed with psychiatric illness and those not so diagnosed with respect to the survival rate after cancer diagnosis, the team analyzed the dated using logistic and Cox models. They found no evidential association between specific mental disorders of individuals diagnosed with cancer and those devoid of cancer. Nevertheless, they did find that individuals suffering from severe mental disorders such as depression, dementia, and substance abuse were more inclined to a diminished survival rate after a cancer diagnosis versus the general population. A modest but telling result in their findings suggested that the relationship between mental disorders and cancer mortality is substantially reckoned with based on differences in the survival rate following a cancer diagnosis rather than the result of a delayed diagnosis of cancer.

As has been discussed earlier in this review of literature, the distinctions between serious mental illness and severe mental illness have yet to be settled within the psychiatric community. However, these terms are commonly used interchangeably essentially characterize the same disorders (see Glossary of Terms). There is still another less highly developed descriptive term for mental illness, i.e., Common Mental Disorders (CMDs), which has been proposed to be inclusive of points of depression and anxiety falling outside the parameters of SMIs (both serious and severe). Often, cancer patients experience an on-going bout with CMDs such that the psychiatric oncologists have chosen to explore the effectiveness of certain psychiatric drugs in the treatment of outpatients suffering from cancer. Unfortunately and owing to the lower level of oncological concern for cancer patients not actually suffering from severe or serious mental disorders, CMDs have been more or less side stepped in terms of research. Flavio Hiroshi Shirama of the University of Sao Paulo, however, has been joined by a clinical staff of oncologists from Brazilian medical research centers to focus precisely upon this under-served field of research (Shirama, Silva, Santos, et al., 2019). The intent of this distinguished panel of researchers in oncological practice was to focus upon the identification of factors which are linked with psychiatric drugs in the treatment of outpatients with cancer suffering from common mental disorders (CMDs).

This Brazilian team of medical researchers called attention to three fundamental factors about the situation of cancer treatment, viz., the high rate of cancer generally throughout Brazil (not unlike the global reality), the high level of common mental disorders (CMDs) found in the treatment of cancer patients, and the overall practice of using psychiatric drugs in the treatment of such patients without clinical evidence of their measurable effectiveness. Therefore, this team of medical researchers have called for a systematic assessment of these psychiatric drugs commonly used in spite of the absence of verifiable effectiveness in the treatment of cancer patients suffering from and being treated for common mental disorders. The aim of this monumental project was to identify these drugs, their prevalence in the treatment of CMDs by oncologists, and to identify factors linking common mental disorders with the use of psychotropic medication in the treatment of cancer outpatients.

Using a cross-sectional study with descriptive correlational design which had been developed in the chemotherapy department of a specialized cancer hospital in Brazil, the team chose to use both the Self-Reporting Questionnaire (SRQ-20) as well as structured questionnaires developed by the team itself. In this limited database of 403 cancer respondents, just over 30% manifested CMD symptoms and just over 25% used some form of psychotropic medication. They found that common mental disorders were most frequently linked to gender, education, family income, psychotropic use and cancer surgery whereas psychotropic use was most commonly linked to gender, employment status, cancer surgery, and treatment period of the patient's cancer as well as other general health considerations. The team found through the use of logistic regressions that patients with CMD, were linked commonly in gender and various physical health conditions whereas patients using psychotropic medication most often were linked to gender and employment status. They called for more focused research on the relationship of CMD and psychiatric medication to get a more accurate picture of the national situation.

Health care professionals have known for a long time, indeed, probably always, that there is a disparity between access and quality of medical care and the socio-economic level of the patient. A further factor in evaluating these disparities is that of the linkage between countries of high and low income levels. The refinement of this matrix of variables was developed by Ora Nakash of the school of psychology at the Interdisciplinary Center in Herzliya, Israel, and a full complement of researchers interested particularly in working with data provided by the World Mental Health Surveys (WMHS). Treatment gaps based on these variables affecting comorbidity of common mental disorders (CMDs) constituted the specific focus of this study based on data provided by the WMHS of 13 high-income and 11 low-middle-income countries. The 66,387 participants were divided into three categories, viz., those with active cancer N=357, cancer survivors N=1,373, and cancer-free respondents N=64,657. In order to establish the common mental disorders prevalence rate, the World Health Organization/Composite International Diagnostic Interview was employed by this research team. To complete the thoroughness of this data analysis, each respondent was questioned regarding their mental health service utilization during the previous 12 months of the study. The actual cancer status of each respondent was based on a self-report of physician's diagnosis. Nationality, income, and prevalence rates of the respondents constituted the fundamental tripartite research focus of this massive databased study.

The research team was able to determine that over the twelve-month period of inquiry there was a prevalence rate of common mental disorders (CMDs) registered at a higher occurrence among active cancer patients (18.4%) than among cancer-free respondents (13.3%). A similar pattern was identified among both high-income and low-middle-income countries while respondents with active cancer with reportable CMDs during the previous 12 months saw some 59% seeking services for self-reported mental health problems. CMD patients using mental health services based on cancer status was only slightly different among the two income classifications with the highest utilization rate being among active cancer patients, somewhat lower among survivors, and lowest among cancer-free respondents. This study confirmed the disparity between active cancer patients with a higher CMD rate than the other classifications as well as a higher treatment gap which suggests that cancer treatment institutions should take account of both factors.

As with any seriously life-threatening illness sustained over time, there are essentially three factors involved, viz., the patient, the patient's significant others, and the health care professionals involved in the overall care of the patient. A major exacerbating component of quality care of a cancer patient is when the patient is also suffering from a mental illness. Though there are anecdotal references to the relationship of mental illness and cancer care, there is a disturbing lack of databased studies as noted in Millman and colleagues at the School of Nursing and Midwifery of the Queen's University Belfast in the UK (Millman, et al., 2016). Any serious address to a void in the refinement of patient care must always be tied to databased studies rather than just editorial surmises. Millman and colleagues set out to explore this phenomenon of the relationship of cancer care and serious mental illness focusing upon the experience of the three relevant members of this matrix, namely, the patient, the patient's family, and the health care professionals providing oversight for each case.

In anticipation of future databased studies and in preparation for an assessment of the relationship between mental illness and the variant quality of cancer care and resulting outcome, the team made a specific point of focusing upon the phenomenon of comorbidity leading to earlier deaths of this matrix of cancer patients with severe mental illness. Previous studies addressing these issues, unfortunately, relied almost exclusively upon specifically healthcare professionals to the exclusion of both the patient and their family support group. This team relied upon a qualitative exploration of such patients of interest involving 35 semi-structured interviews of three categories of respondents, viz., adults with a cancer diagnosis suffering from a serious mental illness, the social support and care providers, and the designated healthcare professionals. These recorded interviews were semi-structured and digitally recorded.

The intent in this projected research project was to direct the questioning specifically to the experience of the respondents having cancer with serious mental illness. Also, such questioning was intended for those individuals providing social support for such respondents with this designated comorbidity. A framework analysis was anticipated as the *modus operandi* and research Ethics Committee and Trust Research & Development approval was a prerequisite to launching this study. Six individuals with experience in dealing with either cancer or mental illness constituted a functioning steering committee that offered feedback and verified the respondents' self-reported information. Owing to the generally recognized scarcity of genuine research data on such individuals with this comorbidity, the intention of this research team was to distribute their findings to relevant professional communities and sources of information in hopes of providing a better support mechanism for this cohort and the professionals serving in their care.

Recognizing that there is a high prevalence of mental illness in cancer patients generally, Susane Kuhnt of the Department of Medical Psychology's section on Psychosocial Oncology at the University Medical Center in Leipzig, Germany, was joined by a cadre of colleagues at that medical center all interested in the prevalence rates of mental disorders over a period of between 12-months and lifetime in cancer patients (Kuhnt, Brahler, Faller, et al., 2016). Being on the staff of the medical center's Department of Medical Psychology and

Sociology specializing in psychosocial oncology (aka psychiatric oncology), this team was focused upon the need for planning psycho-oncological interventions as well as providing services which have been tailored to the particular needs of the various types of cancers within the general population. The challenge early in this databased study was the need to actually determine to what extent variously identified emotional and psychological problems actually conform to accepted definitions of mental disorders. Using a database of 2,141 patients classified into three groupings, i.e., outpatient, inpatient, and rehabilitation environments identified as overall 12-month prevalence (12MP) and lifetime prevalence (LTP), the study employed a standardized computer-assisted Composite International Diagnostic Interview (CIDI-O) developed specifically for cancer patients with identifiably diagnostic mental disorders with differing tumor entities and stages of development.

What the team found was fascinating in that the comparison and contrast between the 12MP and LTP patients proved, contrary to expectations, less easily predictable and less similar than pre-data analysis had suggested. Of the 12MP patients the mental disorder was measured at 39.4% with anxiety disorders measured at 15.8% and mood disorders at 12.5%. The percentages continued to decline such that somatoform disorders were at 9.5%, nicotine dependence at 7.3%, disorders due to general medical conditions at 3.7% and 1.1% due to alcohol dependence.

On the other hand, what these researchers found was that in the case of lifetime prevalence of mental disorders among the study group of 2,141 patients, 56.3% of these individuals suffered from a diagnosable mental disorder with 24.1% suffering from an anxiety disorder, 20.5% from mood disorders, 19.9% from various somatoform disorders, 18.2% from nicotine dependence, 6.4% from alcohol dependency, 4.5% from general medical conditions, and less than 1% from identifiable eating disorders.

A brief statistical comparison between the 12-month prevalence patients and the lifetime prevalence patients demonstrated clearly that the LTP faired consistently better that the 12MP in that the percentage variance between the LTP and 12MP was at 70% for overall mental disorders with 65% and 60% respectively for anxiety disorders and mood disorders. Somatoform disorders and nicotine dependency variant was 40% and 40% respectively. The variances were accounted for in the team's recommendations, based on the high prevalence in cancer patients with a mental disorder, such that provisions for continuous psychiatric oncological support is called for in the case of inpatient as well as outpatient care.

From the early days of oncological research related to mental health there has been a generally held conviction that psychiatric comorbidities are commonly present among cancer patients but at this time very little databased research had actually been attempted. Of particular absence was a verifiable correlation between the increase in mental disorders linked to a cancer diagnosis such that a standardized generalization could be anticipated. Donghao Lu of the Karolinski Institutet in Stockholm, Sweden, was joined by colleagues within the Institutet's medical staff of the Orebro University with the intention of tracking this correlation (D. Lu, Andersson, Fall, et al., 2016). The focus was based upon a nationwide matched cohort study in Sweden tracing the relationship between a clinical diagnosis of a mental illness before and after a cancer diagnosis for the purpose of attempting to determine whether or not and/or to what extent, if at all, there would be a measurable correlation between the relationship of a cancer diagnosis with a mental disorder diagnosis. At the time of this databased study there had not been a reported attempt at such a study. This Institutet study was based on a ten year cohort study from 1.1.2001 to 12.31.2010 of the health register of the Swedish population.

The challenge faced by Lu and colleagues was elevated owing to the size of the cancer population of over 300,000 amidst a cancer-free population of over three million. Using the time-varying hazard ratios (HRs), the research team categorized the cohort into the first clinical diagnosis of mental disorders marked from 2 years prior to the cancer diagnosis throughout the diagnosed period and 10 years following the diagnosis. They adjusted the data for age, sex, calendar period, and educational level and, to offer a more refined assessment, they included a consideration of patients receiving psychiatric medications during the 2008-2009 period. Based on year of birth and sex, there were 304,118 patients with cancer and 3,041,174 cancer-free individuals selected randomly from the Swedish population. Just under half of the patients assessed were female and the median age at the time of diagnosis for cancer was 69 years. What proved of real interest to the team was the fact that after about 10 months prior to a cancer diagnosis, the rate of mental disorders actually increased and peaked during the first week following the cancer diagnosis but commenced decreasing significantly reporting an elevated status for a decade after the initial diagnosis. Non-melanoma skin cancer was the only type of cancer whose elevated rate remained constant but consistently remained constant for cancers which presented a poor prognosis. Psychiatric medications increased from the first months prior to diagnosis and maintained a continuous use with a peak 3 months following the initial diagnosis.

The findings in this massive databased study were striking and somewhat troubling to the healthcare community. Patients who were diagnosed with cancer, for example, actually had an increased risk of several common mental illnesses a full year prior to the initial diagnosis. The data demonstrated a call for an integrated psychological management protocol for cancer care patients and a clarion call for what they called "vigilance" for monitoring various mental disorders from the outset of a cancer diagnosis.

An enduring concern within the oncological research community is the need for a linking of types of cancer with types of mental illness. This constitutes a major focus of research owing to the extremely complicated nature of the available data relevant to this specialized interest. Within that matrix is a particular interest in the relationship between cancer and schizophrenia as upwards of 1% of the world's general population suffers from this particular mental illness. The linkage of cancer to this illness is further exacerbated by the fact that schizophrenic patients have nearly a 20% shorter life span than the general public. By combining data relative to the prevalence of schizophrenia and cancer, this packaging justifies an intense effort at understanding the nature of the linkage. Taiwanese oncologists under the leadership of Frank H-C Chou of the Department of Community Psychiatry at the Kaohsiung Municipal Kai-Syuan Psychiatric Hospital in Taiwan was joined by several colleagues in Taiwan to address specifically this linkage and, if possible, its causes (Chou, Tsai, Wu, Shen, 2016). A side panel of concern recognized by this research team was the realization that this specific topic of cancer and schizophrenia linkage is fundamentally controversial.

The starting point for their research project was that of an address to previous research publications which had shown that cancer patients suffering from schizophrenia experience earlier mortality as compared to the general cancer population. In the absence of verifiable proof of an identifiable causal relationship, there are various suggestions such as the possibility that a lower cancer screening rate coupled with a lack of effective treatment might constitute the matrix within which a causal relationship might be discovered. Studies show that there are three categories of factors which might be contributory, i.e., *patient factors* such as poor lifestyle, passive attitudes towards treatment, and a comorbidity, *physician factors* such as physician bias towards mental illness' relevance to cancer care, and *hospital administration factors* such as intrinsic stigma and discrimination intrinsic within the healthcare delivery system (and staffing) itself. Recognizing this tripartite constellation of potential contributing factors, this research team suggests that further study is clearly called for and should address such issues as a comprehensive view of previously published research on the topic, a concentration on the differentiation of specific types of cancer, and they suggested improvement methods of assessment and treatment.

Rather adventurously, this research team under the leadership of Chou suggested that in light of the need to reduce the early mortality rate of cancer patients suffering from schizophrenia, it might prove beneficial to implement or address five specific improvements, viz., (1) increasing the screening rate for schizophrenic patients facilitating early detection and treatment; (2) offer effective treatment and rehabilitation in a timely and convenient manner; (3) seek to increase the quality of detection of patients' psychiatric symptoms and cognitive impairment; (4) a general commitment by the medical community to develop and promote healthy lifestyles particularly among the most vulnerable; and (5) put forth concerted effort to reduce the general stigma of schizophrenia entertained by the public. Reduction in the care and treatment of cancer patients with schizophrenia must be an enduring responsibility of the medical community if these glaring disparities are to be addressed and corrected.

Recognized within the psychiatric community is the challenge of proffering a universally accepted definition of key mental health terms. The history of psychiatric practice from the earliest days in the 20th century is characterized by definitional controversy, disputes, rancor, and misperceptions regarding key terms in diagnostic assessment and treatment of mental illness. Such terms as psychosis, insanity, psychopathology, dementia, manic depression, etc. all have a long and convoluted history of use and misuse within the profession. Such is not the case with the competing terms of "severe" versus "serious" mental illness but time will tell whether or not and to what extent there will emerge a universally accepted definitional distinction between the two or if one term will win out over the other for the purpose of simplification of diagnostic assessment. In the meantime, a distinguished panel of Danish oncologists from Aarhus University under the leadership of A. Toender has produced a monumentally important national study of the Danish population with data provided by the National Centre for Register-Based Research (Toender, Munk-Olsen, Estergaard, Larsen, et al., 2018). Rather than calling any attention to the tempest in a tea pot regarding the definitional issue of "severe" versus "serious," Toender and team chose the high road by focusing upon the relational impact which inevitably exists between mental illness and the diagnostic stages of cancer and mortality rates. These issues had been a topic of conversation for a number of years but not until this study was there anything like a comprehensive assessment of the data related to this relationship issue. Thanks to Toender and his distinguished panel of leading research oncologists, a significant contribution was made by this research project to a deeper understanding of this relationship.

Because there is statistical verification that a high level of mortality occurs within the individual population suffering from severe mental illness (SMI), the tendency is to account for this excess mortality by attributing the causal factors to physical comorbidity and even suboptimal health care practices without, however, further verification as to whether or not there is a linkage between cancer deaths and psychotic disorders. Realizing that cancer death has an measurable prevalence throughout the world, the team was fully cognizant of the fact that tumor stage at the time of diagnosis constitutes a high level predictor rate for mortality. Therefore, the team set out to study more closely the cancer incidence within the Danish population focusing on the cancer stage at the time of diagnosis and the resulting mortality rate of individuals suffering from severe mental illness as compared to individuals who die of cancer not having a severe mental illness.

The research team concentrated their efforts in a study of the entire Danish population with data provided by the national registry for the 35 year period from 1978 to 2013. To get at the possible causal relationship between cancer and mental illness, the research team took a look at the cancer rate within the national population which resulted ultimately in mortality classification of these subjects by disease stages of those individual rates of death who had a severe mental illness and those who did not. A standard industry-wide procedure was the use of the Cox regression for estimating incidence ratio rates (IRR) with mortality ratio rates (MRR), grouping the cases of cancer using major etiological factors. An interesting (and unexplained) gender distinction in this study found that whereas the rate of cancer among women with and without severe mental illness hardly varied, with men the rate of cancer of those with severe mental illness was actually lower than men with cancer and no registered severe mental illness.

Finally, whereas the overall mortality rate of cancer patients registered higher for those with a diagnosed severe mental illness, the rate was lower for cancer patients without SMI. Even when stratified by tumor size and stage of development including etiological records, the incidence rates and mortality rates were similar across the full cohort spectrum. The team was quick to point out that they did not come to any clarity as to the reason(s) why they found lower cancer rates among men with severe mental illness(SMI) compared to men without a severe mental illness and the same was more or less true for women in both categories as well, i.e., with and without SMI. They did find without explanation the fact that higher mortality rates were found in both sexes with SMI and, therefore, they were able to call for more study based on the data gathered in this national study of the Denmark population.

In recognition of the fact that cancer hospitalizations are on the rise internationally, there is a growing interest in studying the relationship between diagnostic assessment of cancer patients who are admitted at the time with identified mental disorders with particular attention to the emotional distressed experienced by a patient at the time of diagnosis, the relevance of the mental illness, and the significance of hospitalization. Whether or not and/or to what extent a cancer diagnosis of a patient suffering from a mental illness has upon the duration of hospitalization (both the economic as well as the institutional impact) is a question which has been most frequently overlooked in oncology research. Jianwei Zhu of the Karolinska Institutet in Stockholm (Sweden) was joined by several colleagues specifically to examine the relationship of hospitalization, mental illness, and a cancer diagnosis (Zhu, Sjolander, Fall, et al., 2018).

A universally recognized standard procedure (Cox model) to estimate hazard ratios (HRs) with a predicable 95% confidence interval rating (CIs) was used by the research team employing a clinical diagnosis of stress-linked mental disorders measured from 90 days before through to 90 days after a diagnosis of cancer occurred. This research project constituted a national study with a cohort of 218,508 cancer patients who were diagnosed from 2004-2009 in Sweden. The team followed these patients from 90 days following the cancer diagnosis through to 2010. After analyzing total hospitalization admissions initially, the team then divided the cohort into three common admission classifications including external injuries, infections, and cardiovascular diseases. Of the total cohort of 218,508 cancer patients, the team found that 4,105 of the patients had received a diagnosis of stress-related mental disorders at the time of the cancer diagnosis and registered a 35% increase in the rate of hospitalizations during the follow-up period including both admissions for external injuries, infections, and cardiovascular diseases. Based on the overall findings of this databased study, the team concluded that individuals diagnosed with cancer who were suffering from a mental disorder just prior to or immediately following the diagnosis of cancer were much more likely to experience hospitalization due to a major comorbidity of cancer. The team of researchers was eager to emphasize the importance of vigilance in monitoring such patients before, during, and following the diagnostic process.

As we have been discussing the literature over the past four years regarding the range of research in oncology, a major initiative at the Sloan-Kettering Cancer Institute in New York undertaken by Dr. Jimmy Holland in the 1970s led to an international movement focusing upon the psychosocial spectrum of cancer care designed specifically as a compliment and aid to medical oncology (Morgan, 2023). This movement, embodied in the distinguished international publication, *Psychooncology*, has elevated the research topic of the psychosocial spectrum embodied in the life of the cancer patient such that the collaborative efficacy of bio-medical and psychosocial components of cancer has become a normative domain assumption in all meaningful assessment and treatment modalities. (In the Appendix, we have listed 25 major cancer research centers around the world which now include psychiatric oncology as a central component of overall health care). Combining these two complimentary spheres of research and treatment with an interest in the psychiatric disorders and mental illnesses so common among cancer patients and we have produced a tripartite constellation of medical, social, and behavioral factors all evidenced commonly among cancer patients. (A listing of over 100 scholarly periodicals addressing issues in cancer research is provided in the Appendix.)

A distinguished team of internationally recognized oncologists under the leadership of P. U. Prakash Saxena of the Katurba Medical College in Karnataka, India, was mobilized to do a comprehensive assessment of the broad range of assessments and modalities of treatments of cancer patients suffering concurrently from diagnosed mental disorders. This team launched their databased research based on the universally recognized reality that cancer is one of the most pernicious and leading causes of disability and their domain assumption centered upon the realization that the psychosocial character affecting the cancer patient's capacity to navigate life's daily demands comprises a cluster of mental illnesses composed of anxiety, depressive disorders, and somatization. In their quest to identify and circumscribe the broad spectrum of psychiatric disorders commonly found in cancer patients, they set out to locate and delineate the nature of the association between what they identified as sociodemographic variables and treatment modalities linked to the range of psychological issues facing many cancer patients.

At the Medical College in Kamataka (India), this team of researchers conducted a cross-sectional study of cancer patients who were at the time receiving treatment. In an effort to produce databased results of this study of anxiety and depression screening, the team employed the Patient Health Questionnaire (PHQ) for somatization, anxiety and depression screeners which is essentially a pre-validated standardized questionnaire usually coupled with the PHQ-9, the generalized anxiety disorder 7, and the PHQ-15 which combines with a panic measurement from initial data provided by the PHQ. The result was a well-developed and refined questionnaire which was then administered to patients undergoing treatment at the time and later subjected to a rigorous assessment by the research team. Using the SPSS version 16, the project focused on the linkage between identified relevant variables which were then scrutinized through the employment of the Chi-square test. They found that a range of psychiatric morbidities characterized the cancer patients in this study. These cancer patients were actually suffering from depression and the team discovered that there existed a significant linkage between the cancer patients in the study and their residential addresses showing an elevated rate of radiotherapy utilization.

The findings of this databased study and the conclusions drawn by the research team were extensive and insightful. They discovered, for example, that emotional, psychiatric, and mental problems generally were elevated with cancer patients living in rural areas of the country and among female cancer patients somewhat higher than among male cancer patients. Of real significance was the discovery that the highest levels of anxiety and somatization existed among cancer patients in Stage II of development with depression highest in Stage IV. They further found that the highest levels of anxiety existed among patients undergoing chemotherapy treatment at the time and that this particular treatment modality also saw patients who were receiving chemotherapy as well as radiotherapy having a higher level of somatization. Depression proved to be highest among those cancer patients who were receiving radiotherapy treatment.

Two fundamental components of overall cancer care constitute a duality of complementing responsibility and compliance, namely, on the part of the patient who is willing (and able) to comply with cancer care directives and on the part of the medical care team to explain and insure compliance of the patient with the protocol directives. Both patient and clinicians must embrace their mutually interlocking responsibilities and when it comes to patients who are comorbid with both cancer and mental illness, the challenge is exponentially greater than otherwise. A number of databased researches have addressed this overall problem of securing compliance with cancer care directives for patients suffering from a mental illness but more work needs to be done to identify those modalities of care and treatment which gain the highest compliance rates. Zhihong Li of the School of Basic Medical Sciences at Lanzhou University in China has put together a team of likeminded research oncologists with the intention of measuring the effectiveness of what is called Acceptance and Commitment Therapy (ACT) using a systematic review and meta-analysis of Randomized Controlled Trials (RCT) as reported in a key research-based article (Li, Li, Guo, Li, Yang, 2021).

The care and treatment of cancer patients has always involved a component of emotional compliance with the protocol of care but the recognition and acceptance of the situation of a cancer diagnosis is greatly influenced by the awareness by the patient of the disease itself. The psychosocial spectrum of cancer care, though recognized at various levels for many decades of care protocol, there has been limited quantitative studies of the effectiveness of various methods of care and treatment. Li and colleagues set out to examine more closely the actually measurable effectiveness of what is called Acceptance and Commitment Therapy (ACT) applicable specifically to the treatment of cancer in patients suffering from mental illness. In the absence of consistent studies of ACT and the growing need for documented verification of its effectiveness (or not), this team of Chinese oncologists have initiated a substantial databased study of the issue beginning with 10 database studies which they searched in publications using such search tools as mental health, cancer, and Randomized Controlled Trials (RCT). Then, to assure objectivity, they appointed two researchers who were directed to independently screen the extracted data from the publications judging the quality of those studies and their databases.

Of the 877 cancer patients identified in 17 RCTS, they were judged of low quality compared with the control group whereas the ACT studies showed a higher level of quality outcomes following treatment covering a span of 1 to 3 months and again 3 months to 6 months. In these assessments, depression, anxiety, quality of life, psychological distress, and stress were all assessed. Acceptance and Commitment Therapy was linked with psychological flexibility and did not show signs of linkage with a reduction of fear of treatment but even after 6 months of follow-up, such mental issues as depression, anxiety, quality of life, and stress continued to be of significance. They did find that after an extended period of time the effects of ACT showed that psychological flexibility (1-3 months) actually decreased and fear (1-6 months) also decreased. The research led the team to conclude that though ACT can demonstrate an effective contribution as a treatment component of cancer care owing to the fact that it was shown in these studies to actually reduce or alleviate depression, anxiety, stress, fear, yet improving the quality of life, there is still very much a need for further databased studies of ACT assessed over an extended period of time and that high quality RCTs are called for in more reliable findings might be discovered.

A common and baffling occurrence in cancer therapeutic treatment is that of non-adherence to prescribed protocols. Some types of cancer are more negatively impacted by non-compliance to medication procedures than others. A particularly pernicious complications has to do with breast cancer patients suffering from mental illness who fail to adhere to endocrine therapy protocols. The prominence of this problem constitutes the focus of Cole B. Haskins of the College of Public Health at the University of Iowa where a team of medical researchers were joined by other professionals who set as their research agenda a study of the impact pre-diagnosed mentally ill patients suffering from breast cancer experience when failing to adhere to set endocrine therapy procedures (Haskins, McDowell, Carnahan, et al., 2019). Based on established documented clinical studies of patients with estrogen receptor positive (ER+) breast cancer who commonly fail to comply with endocrine therapies even though these therapies have a positive track record of efficacy, this research team initiated their research using a national cancer cohort representative roster of cancer patients suffering from specific mental illnesses in order to assess this non-compliant behavioral response to endocrine therapy adherence.

The particulars of the study group were refined closely based on data secured from the SEER-Medicare database which, in this research project, included 21,894 women over 67 years of age having had their first surgically treated state I-IV ER+breast cancer covering a period from 2007 to 2013. Participation in the study was restricted to cancer patients who enjoyed a fee-for-service Medicare Parts A and B for at least three years prior to the diagnosis and 18 or more months following the diagnosis. This also included patients with continuous Part D of Medicare for four months or more prior to and 18 months or more following the diagnosis. Within the context of analyzing endocrine therapy adherence and discontinuation based on longitudinal linear and Cox regression models, the team limited their study to women with a mental illness which had occurred during the previous three years prior to the onset of the cancer being treated.

Of the mental illnesses evaluated in this study were primarily unipolar depression (11%), anxiety (9.5%), and non-schizophrenia psychosis and dementias (both at 4.6%) for these four disorders were the most commonly seen in the study. The team identified 80% of the female cancer patients as having had endocrine therapies and of those with at least 12 months of treatment, nearly 30% were actually non-adherent with over 25% discontinuing treatment. A surprisingly hopeful finding in this study was that cancer patients suffering from dementia as well as bipolar depression/psychotic/schizophrenia disorders actually registered a lower adjusted initiation probability during the first year of follow-up whereas patients without these designated disorders did not. Disappointing was the finding that cancer patients subject to substance abuse or anxiety disorders failed more commonly to discontinue endocrine therapy for at least a year after adjustment with a registered lower adherence rate than otherwise.

This research team was able to verify that upwards of 25% of female cancer patients who received Medicare benefits registered a diagnosed mental illness prior to an invasive breast cancer diagnosis and treatment. The concern throughout was that of the abandonment of treatment by the high risk cancer patient suffering from a mental illness. It remains the overall research concern for even though there has been a slightly measurable reduction in the rates of initiation, adherence, and discontinuation of treatment, endocrine therapy compliance is persisting as a suboptimal, unnecessarily worsening event leading to increased risk of mortality.

The cross-over in research between what is relevant to the medical care and treatment of diagnosed cancer patients and the nature and relevance of insurance claims is a fascinating yet only marginally studied relationship. To focus upon one particular type of cancer, namely, head and neck cancer (HNC) relative to its relationship to survival rates and recurrence rates constituted the impetus for the large databased research project conducted at the College of Medicine of the Pennsylvania State University under the leadership of Ji Hyae Lee and several of his institutional colleagues (Lee, Ba, Liu, Leslie, et al., 2019).

Though there have been several databased studies showing that Mental Health Disorders (MHDs) are commonly linked with a 5-year survival and recurrence rate for cancer patients suffering from HNC, unfortunately there has to-date been a shortage of verifiable replications of large databased research. Lee and colleagues set out to address this shortage of replication using data provided by records provided by a large insurance claim database.

Employing a retrospective cohort study based on data provided by the MarketScan database from January 1, 2005 to December 31, 2014, the team sought to identify the common presence of mental health disorders in cancer patients suffering from HNC with the intent of linking that information with both survival and recurrence data based on insurance claim data. The whole study was based on medical records of 52,641 HNC cancer patients during the designated time span. Owing to the size of the initial cohort number and in an attempt to avoid errors caused by patients with a pre-existing HNC diagnosis and those with insufficiently completed data records, the team limited the final cohort to patients who had not been diagnosed for 12 months prior to the beginning of the study. They limited their data analysis to patients covering the time frame from February 20, 2017 through January 22, 2019.

Using standardized tests for independent findings, the team sought to assess the common occurrence of mental health disorders both before and after the diagnosis of head and neck cancer. The team developed a multivariable logistic regression test using Adjusted Adds Ratios (AORs) comparing the occurrence of MHDs in oral cavity cancer patients with those suffering from other types of cancer located in the head and neck area of the body. Cohort participants taken from the 52,641 were commonly limited to patients averaging 51 years of age (58.5% men), patients aged 55 to 64 years of age (46.6%), and patients from the South at 40.3% were most commonly suffering from HNC. Furthermore, oral cavity cancer constituted 40.4% of the cohort which was the most common type seconded by cancer of the oropharynx (nearly 20%) and larynx (just over 15%). Cancer found in the trachea was measurably elevated based on the MHD as compared with other oral cavity cancer. Significantly mental health disorders of patients suffering from head and neck cancers increased nearly 30% as compared with a 20% instance prior to the cancer diagnosis. Of particular relevance to insurance claims was the fact that women and patients having a record of tobacco and alcohol abuse showed a measurably higher rate of mental health disorders following the diagnosis of head and neck cancer.

The National Survey on Drug Use and Health shows a national average of almost 18% with the team's records showing nearly 21% baseline for MHD prevalence among their cohort studied with a near 30% increase in MHDs following a cancer diagnosis. Of particular note was the fact that cancer patients (especially women) with tobacco and alcohol abuse histories were especially vulnerable to a diagnosis of mental health disorders. The team showed conclusively that there is a direct linkage between head and neck cancer patients and an increase occurrence of mental health disorders following treatment as compared to the national population.

Much of that which has occupied over time in this study of research during the past decades has focused upon cancer and mental illness as an area of problematic diagnosis and treatment. What has not been considered are those individuals who have continued to thrive during a diagnosis of cancer without either having or developing a psychiatric disorder. Very little attention has been given to this category of patients though clearly there is statistical evidence that such individuals do exist and beyond surviving actually thrive in the midst of their cancer. Esme Fuller-Thomson and Keri J. West have chosen to seek out data relative to those individuals over the age of 50 years whom they characterize as "flourishing" amidst their cancer diagnosis while maintaining what they have characterized as a "complete mental health" status (Fuller-Thomson, West, 2019). Both researchers are from the University of Toronto working in the fields of social work, aging, and community medicine.

Psychiatric oncologists direct their research attention to the psychosocial spectrum of cancer care and in the absence of any documented and verified biochemical causal relationship between a cancer and mental illness, the attention has been directed to the life situation of the patient who may have a psychiatric disorder in an attempt to determine when the relationship appeared and the factors contributing to it. The focus in the Fuller-Thomson and West study is upon the cancer patient characterized as having complete mental health (CMH) manifesting optimal functionality devoid of any detectable psychopathology. The researchers employed a secondary database from the nationally representative 2012 Canadian Community Health Survey-Mental Health and using a bivariate and logistic regression analysis in their efforts to estimate the CMH odds ratio among community participants aged 50 years and older. This group of participants were divided into those with current cancer (n=438), those with previous cancer (n=1,174), and those without any history of cancer (n=9,279).

The challenge for the research project's integrity centered round a viable definition of "complete mental health" such that the definitional parameters were set within a tripartite arrangement of (1) the absence of any traceable mental illness, addictions, or any suicidal thoughts within the past year; (2) a reported daily happiness or satisfaction with life during the immediately preceding month; and (3) a self-reported psychosocial well-being. Granted the qualitative nature of this self-characterization, the research clearly was required to take full cognizance of a range of what the research team called "control variables" which included socio-demographics, health behaviors, and present physical health of the respondent as well as a lifetime history of mental illness or childhood maltreatment.

Within the scope of these pre-set parameters used to establish the definitional range of this study of CMH, the study focused on adults aged 50 years or older having cancer at the time of the study. These individuals showed much less prevalence of complete mental health (66%+) to those individuals who reported previously having cancer (77%+) and those with no cancer history at all (76%+). The thoroughness of this study is reflected in the researchers identifying 17 variables which informed their analysis of respondents wherein they found that the chances of complete mental health of patients presently having cancer was significantly lower than individuals without any cancer. However, for individuals who had a history of cancer, the chances that they might be designated complete mental health subjects were measurably higher for White married females as well as older respondents but particularly for those individuals who were located within a higher socioeconomic status within society having no history of childhood physical abuse, substance abuse, depression or any anxiety disorder. Their final conclusion based on these data led them to suggest that there is a measurably higher level of resilience among cancer survivors for individuals who previously had cancer had a similar rate of CMH among individuals never having had cancer.

An abiding research and clinical practice issue which has always characterized the treatment of cancer patients with a diagnosed mental illness has to do with to what extent there is a measurable and identifiable linkage between cancer and mental health such that predictions with respect to treatment protocols and outcomes can be documented. Not uncommonly, there is a clash between the treatment of a cancer patient and the patient's own state of mental health such that the patient's serious mental illness and psychiatric disorder constitute a major stumbling block in the overall care and treatment of the patient. Amy Hemmington of the Psychology and Social Work Department of the Counties Manukau Health of Auckland (NZ) has been joined by several of her colleagues from the University of Auckland and the Counties Manukau Health Department to focus specific research on the problematics of the anticipated collision between mental illness and cancer care (Hemmington, Huang, Coomarasamy, et al. 2020). The special focus was upon a carefully constructed inquiry into the actual factors allowing for an outcome prediction of results from cancer patients with a mental illness history.

Hemmington and colleagues began their inquiry with a clear understanding that individuals with a diagnosably serious mental illness or psychiatric disorder are not more inclined to receive a cancer diagnosis than is the general public. However, records show that these individuals are more likely to do less well in terms of outcome of assessment and treatment of cancer. Therefore, this team of researchers chose to focus on whether or not a cancer patient with a history of mental illness (as determined by a history of contact with mental health services and psychotropic medications) beyond the demographic and general medical factors actually affect the cancer patient's outcome of treatment. There were 1,652 diagnosed cancer patients provided by the Counties Manukau Health Department covering a period from the first of January of 2016 to the last day of December of that year covering a full 12 months of patient data. The study group was divided into three separate categories, namely, those with no mental health issues, those with a moderate mental health record, and those with a diagnosed serious mental illness or psychiatric disorder.

This original idea of a three-way classification of patients proved most insightful to the research team for they found that cancer patients classified in the second (moderate) and third (serious) group demonstrated a susceptibility to physical comorbidities more than in classification one (no mental illness). Furthermore, they discovered that patients suffering from a serious mental illness were more or less susceptible to having advanced cancer at the time of diagnosis. What proved somewhat surprising was that even though there were no measurable differences in the three groupings regarding the timeframe for treatment and delays, those cancer patients in the third grouping (serious mental illness) were clearly more susceptible to hospitalization and death within the immediate 12 month period following the initial diagnosis. The team did suggest that the recorded differences in mortality could possibly be understood in terms of the more complex clinical situation of the patient such as being older or having other physical comorbidities as well as a later stage of cancer identification. They did find that hospitalization was not linked to any mental health issues.

What clearly was discovered and confirmed in this databased study was that a cancer patient with a personal history of serious mental illness does not do as well as those with moderate mental illness or none at all and what, at the end of the day, may prove indicative of this disparity is the clinical complexities of working with cancer patients with both diagnosed mental and physical comorbidities.

A fundamental field of oncological research linked to psychiatric oncology and the psychosocial spectrum of cancer care is that of the disparities of treatment and survival rates of cancer patients who also have a history of mental illness. Studies consistently show that cancer patients with mental illness who are characterized as having a reduced social life and occupational and functional capacities are particular vulnerable to systemic diagnosis, assessment and treatment disparities. What is missing from databased verification is evidence that the survival rate of these particularly vulnerable cancer patients with mental illness is actually affected by these very disparities of diagnosis and treatment. Laura E. Davis of the Evaluative Clinical Sciences Department of the Sunnybrook Research Institute of Toronto has put together a distinguished team of research-oriented medical professionals from her own institution as well as that of the University of Toronto, Queen's University of Kingston, and the University of Manitoba College of Medicine to focus a specialized inquiry into precisely the issues characterizing this disparity (Davis, Bogner, Coburn, Hanna, et al., 2020). To identify those factors within a mental illness matrix might provide a better understanding of both the survival rate of cancer patients and the on-going effectiveness of cancer care and treatment. However, unless the nature of mental illness is more clearly identified and delineated, the oncology and psychiatric communities are left guessing as to the nature of that relationship.

Covering more than a dozen years of databased records (January 2005 to November of 2018), this tem used the

MEDLINE and PubMed sources for a systematic review and a meta-analysis of observational studies provided by these two major resources. The team appointed two reviewers to evaluate a range of citations which were then incorporated into the study. They chose to define advanced stage cancer as regional or metastatic based on a pre-set classification model in which cancer survival was circumscribed with a definition based on time survived from the initial diagnosis of cancer. While pooling Odd Ratios (ORs) and Hazard Ratios (HRs) in this grouping of research studies, they used the Newcastle-Ottawa bias risk assessment scale as well as Random-effects models employed using the Mantel-Haenszel approach and the generic inverse variance method.

In spite of the thoroughness of their assessment of some 2,381 citations involving 28 studies, this research team found a plethora of flawed methodological missteps in the literature which inevitably reduced the quality of their interpretation of the data resulting in substantial heterogeneity of assessed valuation of their findings. A range of factors influenced the effectiveness of the size of their study including data source selection, definitions of mental illness as well as outcomes and their measurement and predictably an over-adjustment for causal pathway variables. In spite of these limitations identified and articulated by the research team itself, they found that cancer patients manifesting a diagnosed mental disorder had a predictably high susceptibility to advanced stage cancer at the time of diagnosis and, therefore, are more likely to be at risk of a diminished cancer survival rate. Combined with this was the discovery that cancer patients manifesting a more severe mental illness or psychiatric disorder, such as schizophrenia or bi-polar disorder, are subject to a higher rate of cancer disparities. They concluded that a higher quality of research is called for if systemic improvements in the care of psychiatric patients and their support group during cancer diagnosis and follow-up are to occur. Critical gaps inevitably turned up in this review of research covering cancer stages of development from diagnosis to survival for patients suffering from pre-existing mental illness.

A major initiative at the Sloan-Kettering Cancer Institute in New York was undertaken by Dr. Jimmy Holland in the 1970s which led to an international movement focusing upon the psychosocial spectrum of cancer care designed specifically as a compliment and aid to medical oncology (Morgan, 2023). This movement, embodied in the distinguished international publication, *Psychooncology*, has elevated the research topic of the psychosocial spectrum embodied in the life of the cancer patient such that the collaborative efficacy of bio-medical and psychosocial components of cancer has become a normative domain assumption in all meaningful assessment and treatment modalities. Joining this approach to the care of cancer patients with mental health issues was Luigi Grassi of the Institute of Psychiatry in the Department of Biomedical and Specialty Surgical Sciences at the University of Ferrara in Italy. Over the past 20 years he has established himself as a leading voice in psychiatric oncology (Grassi, 2020). In an article published in 2020 in the periodical *Epidemiological Psychiatry* Grassi delineated the issues involved in the linkage of psychiatry and the psychosocial spectrum of cancer care with a special emphasis upon psychiatric oncology as a rightful player in the care of cancer patients. The biomedical side of cancer is attended to by the clinical oncologists but the emotional side of cancer must be attended to with equal commitment by members of the psychiatric and psychotherapeutic professionals working in consort with the entire medical team. To treat cancer as singularly a somatic condition is to overlook the broader range of holistic medicine wherein both the biochemical and psychosocial components of the patient's life are taken into account in the treatment protocol embodied in psychiatric oncology.

Not one to hold back when it comes to developing more advanced approaches to the care and treatment of the cancer patient, Grassi points out that the World Health Organization's epidemiological estimations for new cancer cases in the coming decades including deaths and long-term survivals, there is a crying need for a more aggressive incorporation of the psychosocial care of cancer patients accompanying clinical oncology. Evidence is incontrovertible that upwards of half of all cancer patients also suffering from some manifestation of mental illness and psychiatric disorders including a range of emotional distress signals and a plethora of undiagnosed or unidentified psychosocial conditions which has resulted from the patient's encounter with a cancer diagnosis. Rather than wading into the troubling waters of a possible link between emotional disorders and biochemical imbalance in the cancer patient's somatological state, Grassi has proposed taking a closer look at the relevance of such issues as the diminishment of quality of life in the newly diagnosed patient including such characteristics as a decline in social relationships, longer periods of rehabilitation resulting from newly developed treatments, and a consistent failure of the patient to conscientiously follow treatment protocols.

Continuing to push for the efficacy of psychiatric oncological participation in overall cancer care, Grassi makes a case that in view of the above roster of factors affecting the quality of life of a diagnosed cancer patient it is time for the oncology community worldwide to embrace the IPOS

Standards of Quality Cancer Care which incorporates an awareness of the psychosocial spectrum of cancer care (Morgan, 2023). The argument is that if cancer care is to be holistic, then beyond the five vital signs of health including temperature, blood pressure, pulse, respiratory rate and levels of pain, the medical establishment should embrace the sixth vital sign which is the psychosocial domain of health. Granted the social inequalities of cancer care across the international spectrum including the disparities of organization and utilization of psychiatric oncology, there does exist a range of directives and guidelines regarding screening, assessment and intervention offered for treatment of psychiatric and psychosocial disorders for the overall care of cancer patients. Therefore, Grassi has suggested that both the clinical as well as political agenda of psychiatric oncology should be treated as an indispensable component of a holistic approach to the care and treatment of the cancer patient employing what he labels a "person-centered approach" to the cancer patient, an approach which he calls upon the psychiatric community to endorse and embrace.

A common mistake within the general population is to make uninformed and misinformed observations and to draw conclusions based on such when it comes to general health issues and quite frequently particularly related to cancer. Falsely surmised that cancer is cancer and any observation about the causes of cancer causes is applicable to all types of cancers. In the oncology community, there is a constant struggle to undo these false ideas held in the general public about the nature of cancer and to replace such false notions with a correct understanding of the relevance of the different types of cancer linked to the responsible behavior one takes towards any diagnosis of cancer. This challenge is exacerbated exponentially when the cancer patient is also suffering from a severe mental illness such that correct information and responsible behavior regarding the care of the patient becomes problematic. Further complications beyond mental illness arise over variables such as patient education, age, gender, socioeconomics and residential demographics. What seldom if ever comes within the purview of databased oncology research is the issue of the patient's religious orientation (and this topic we will avoid here anticipating a future major study following publication of this study of cancer and mental illness).

As has already been mentioned, a leading research scholar and published author in this field of enquiry is that of Luigi Grassi of the Department of Neuroscience and Rehabilitation at the University of Ferrara's Institute of Psychiatry in Italy. Joined by a dozen likeminded and credentialed colleagues from his own university as well as that of the University of Michigan in the U.S., Grassi and colleagues set out to better understand the significance of cancer patient knowledge and cancer behavior relative to the level of risk involved for those cancer patients also suffering from severe mental illness (Grassi, Caruso, Biancosino, et al., 2021). Granted the range of patients' knowledge of and behavior toward their own cancer, Grassi and associates were fully cognizant of the wide scope of variant levels of understanding of cancer by the average patient but they were particularly aware of the great disparity of information cancer patients have who are also suffering from a mental illness. This category of patient suffers at a significantly higher rate of risk relative to their behavioral response to their own cancer and the importance of concern for and attention to their own well-being than experienced by patients not suffering from mental illness.

In their concerted effort to come to a better understanding of the nature and function of the knowledge base of the cancer patient including the patient's perception of their own cancer and the risk factors involved in that cancer, this team set out to compare this information deficiency among patients with severe mental illness with cancer patients without a mental illness. Combining a qualitative method of an *ad hoc* semi-structured interview with a quantitative questionnaire of some 17 short true/false responses, the team identified a number of cancer patients (n=185) suffering from a severe mental illness of three types, viz., schizophrenia spectrum disorders, bipolar disorders, and severe personality disorders. They used a gender/age matched control group of primary care attenders and used the interviews and questionnaire to examine the family history of cancer including cancer risk-related lifestyles, personal perception and knowledge of cancer risk factors. They found that nearly half of the study group suffered from schizophrenia spectrum disorders while a third from mood disorders which varied significantly from the control group of primary care attenders (n=173) covering such procedures as lower participation in occult stool blood screening test, Pap smear test and mammography, a higher prevalence of current and past smoking habits; a lower awareness of their own physical symptoms and their understanding of the risks involved in their cancer, a lower physical exercise practicing lifestyle, and a reduced knowledge and understanding of the risk factors involved in having been diagnosed with cancer.

Not surprisingly, the research team found that cancer patients with a diagnosed mental illness experienced an elevated at-risk behavioral matrix for cancer while manifesting a reduced level of concern over their physical health reflecting a minimalist knowledge about cancer risk as compared to the control group. A call for implementation of rigorous screening for cancer among this category of cancer patients was issued by the research team and an appeal for the designing of evidence-based interventionist protocols to minimize cancer risk among cancer patients with severe mental illness.

So much of oncological research focused on cancer care and mortality has historically centered around the patient's response to the scope and nature of diagnosis and treatment. Though this should naturally constitute the lion's share of the research agenda, the characterization of the scope and nature of the professional's perception and practice of caring for the patient must also receive major attention. The importance of this inquiry into the professional care givers' attitudes towards the cancer patient is further complicated with the presence of a severe mental illness in the cancer patient such that the care team must be both cognizant of the nature of the patient's response to the actual cancer as well as to the presence of a psychiatric disorder which inevitably complicates the treatment protocol as well as the care team's assessment of and response to the cancer patient with a mental illness. Tsuyoshi Etoh of the Department of Nursing at the Shimane University Hospital in Japan has chosen to focus a qualitative research project precisely on this duality of cancer and mental illness from the perspective of the oncology health professional and in doing so has put together a distinguished panel of professional oncologists and medical professionals from a range of top Japanese institutions (Etoh, Fujiwara, Yamada, Izumo, et al., 2021). Covering the full spectrum of health care professionals from oncology to psychiatry and nursing, this team of 18 colleagues focused their research agenda on the cancer care of patients with mental illness from the perspective of the caring behavior of the attending professionals overseeing the assessment and treatment of this specialized group of patients.

Disparities and inequities in the care and treatment of cancer patients is well known and documented including such variables as age, gender, socioeconomic status, and education and not least of these relevant variables is that of the cancer patient suffering from a mental disorder. These disparities and inequities manifest themselves at multiple levels from the individual patient and practitioner to institutional and governmental administrative policies such that the study of the delivery system of a medical institution specifically treating cancer patients always proves to be extremely tedious and complicated. Exacerbating these issues is the absence of a consistent and sustained assessment of the professional service staff including particularly the oncologists charged with the care of the cancer patient and the institution responsible for the facilitation of a caring environment. Etoh's team of research professionals chose specifically to address and investigate a full spectrum of issues relevant to the perceptions and perspectives of both the attending personnel such as oncologists and psychiatrists but also of the hosting institutions for cancer care and treatment.

The team identified 754 health care professionals who were asked in an open-ended questionnaire to describe issues they were concerned about regarding the care of cancer patients with mental disorders. These professionals were distributed throughout various medical clinics, designated cancer and psychiatric hospitals as well as various local healthcare/welfare facilities. Of the initially contacted professionals for this study, nearly 60% (439 of 754) actually responded to the qualitative questionnaire identifying some 61 issues categorized into 10 groupings, viz., patient factors;

isolation and lack of support; obstacles to transport; socioeconomic factors; attitudes of psychiatric professionals; medical system of psychiatric hospitals; attitudes of cancer care professionals; medical system of designated cancer hospitals; regional cancer medical systems; and lack of coordination among multidisciplinary healthcare professionals. By assessing these responses, the team was able to propose 48 specific solutions to the problems identified and were delineated into 12 groups of goals. These findings assisted the research team in identifying and delineating exacerbating issues of disparities in the care of cancer patients with a mental illness. They were able to identify a range of issues characterizing not only the patient level of care but that of public policy as well. The urgent need for a broad spectrum of multidisciplinary approaches to the care of cancer patients with mental disorders was evidently applicable to the cancer and psychiatric care professionals involved in treatment protocols such that by the implementation of the suggested solutions there might be a closing of the gap between quality of care and care of the cancer patient with mental disorders. The suggestion by the team was that in addition to being of great value to healthcare practice in Japan, their study might have international relevance.

As has been demonstrated throughout this study of the relationship between cancer and mental illness is the breadth and depth of nomenclature describing mental disorders and psychiatric illnesses. The field is replete with variations on every proposed comprehensive term such that the glossary in this book is crucial to sort out and arrange the significant variations designed to both provide clarity and range of application in such an inquiry. Mental illness, mental disorders, psychiatric illness, psychiatric disorders, emotional dysfunction, etc., as examples and the list goes on. In an attempt to circumscribe the maximum coverage of all variations in the emotional health of a cancer patient, Dorothy Leahy and team have proposed the use of a concept which was imagined to be all inclusive, viz., "significant mental health difficulties (SMHD)." In our glossary, we have ventured a description of this concept relative to mental health which includes a person's emotional, psychological, and social well-being. It affects how an individual thinks, feels, and acts. It also helps determine how a person handles stress, relates to others, and makes healthy choices.

From the School of Psychology at the University of College in Dublin, Dorothy Leahy was joined by colleagues from that institution as well as from the Department of Psychiatry at the Harvard Medical School to focus research attention upon what they chose to characterize as barriers and facilitators to quality cancer care provided for cancer patients suffering from a significant mental health issue by employing a qualitative review and narrative combined method of inquiry (Leahy, Donnelly, Irwin, D'Alton, 2021). Recognizing clearly the disparities reflected in the inequities of cancer care throughout the world reflected in the higher rates of mortality for cancer patients suffering from SMHD as compared to the general population, this team of researchers set out to assess systematically through a review designed to identify, appraise and then synthesize qualitative demonstrations of both patient and clinical barriers to effective cancer screening and treatment protocols for cancer patients suffering from SMHD. To substantiate the relevance of this in-depth research project, they reported that they had engaged in a systematic search using three electronic databases for 2020 and followed that with another search accessing five electronic databases the following year even using a narrative synthesis of relevant articles.

In this study of both patient and clinicians attitudes towards a cancer diagnosis for a patient simultaneously suffering from mental illness, i.e., significant mental health difficulties (SMHD), there was special attention given to the common debilitating factor of stigmatization of the patient by both the patient and the team of health care professionals. Leahy and team studies 133 patients with SMHD and their experiences of cancer care as they reported it and of 102 healthcare professionals and their reported attitudes towards the cancer SMHD patients. They found that a fundamental barrier to cancer care of the patient was linked directly with the patient's uncontrolled psychiatric symptoms reflecting the negative impact that these symptoms carried in the care of the cancer patient. Clinical barriers experienced (and often unfortunately perpetuated) by the attending healthcare professionals had to do with the stigmatization of attitudes towards cancer patients with SMHD resulting too often in the diminishment of the quality and conscientiousness of care given to the patient by both the attending staff as well as the institutional embodiment of these negative attitudes.

A perpetual challenge to oncology health services is avoiding the dangers of a high mortality rate among cancer patients suffering from mental illness. In order to foster a more conscientiously demonstrated positive result from a cancer treatment protocol, the Leahy team placed much emphasis upon the patient's access to quality care and the insistence upon the patient's compliance with treatment directives including the monitoring of controlled psychiatric symptoms. There is clearly an urgent need for a closer collaboration between healthcare professionals working with cancer patients with mental disabilities while paying particular attention to the role of the patient navigator in assuring patient compliance with treatment regiments. The ever present fly in the ointment is that of the mental health stigma not only on the part of the patient but on that of the health care providers as well. Only by doing so will there be any significant improvement in the mortality gap between cancer patients without SMHD and those with SMHD.

During the writing of my book *Cancer and Suicide,* it became crystal clear that there is an information gap between what is known within the psychiatric oncology community and the general public with respect to the relationship between cancer and mental illness. The real danger, of course, is for the general public to assume that cancer can cause mental illness as well as mental illness can cause cancer. Neither of these assumptions are clinically true but the damage to the public mind is enormous particularly as relates to patients suffering from either or both diseases. The importance of educating the public regarding these misperceptions could not be over-emphasized and H. Kim and his two colleagues, K. Kim, and Y. H. Kim, of the Department of Laboratory Medicine at the Pusan National University Hospital in Korea have chosen to address these disparities by examining a range of medical studies from a host of countries using a systematic review and meta-analysis of observational approaches (Kim, Kim, Kim, et al., 2022). The core research task was to delineate in as refined a fashion as possible the complex nature and scope of the linkage between mental illness and cancer in light of the monumental impact this linkage has upon oncology and psychiatric health.

Setting a firm date of October 21, 2020, the researchers examined the Embase and Medline databases including cohort, case-control, and cross-sectional studies which qualified for this examination and analysis. Furthermore, the Newcastle-

Ottawa scale was employed to actually assess the qualitative risk of bias in the examination of published documents and funnel plots were utilized to assess the bias risk across the full spectrum of studies considered. The scope of this database study is reflected in the fact that 58 studies from 16 countries were examined using 30 national databases and 25 million individuals. Cancer patients who displayed psychiatric disorders in this study did not demonstrate an elevated risk of developing cancer but patients with a cancer diagnosis did manifest a substantially elevated risk of developing a mental illness. What also proved most informative relative to mortality was the rate of survival among cancer patients with mental illness shown by cancer occurrence as well as patients with cancer as shown by mental illness occurrence whick were significantly decreased. Based on these findings, the research team suggested that clinical personnel serving in oncology health care facilities should employ cancer screening earlier rather than later in order to anticipate the need for interventions for mentally ill patients receiving cancer treatment. Owing to the elevated rate of deaths among cancer patients with diagnosed mental illness due to unnatural causes such as suicide, homicide, and accidents, attending health care professionals must keep this danger in mind in managing treatment protocols for this classification of patient.

An abiding concern among oncologists, both in research and clinical practice, are the blatant and glaring disparities and inequities in the quality of cancer care around the world contrasted between industrial and developing societies. A further point of concern is the absence of a sustained commitment to clinical research in these developing societies comparable to the high level of sophisticated research in the industrial nations of the world. To launch a robust response to this gap in the treatment of cancer constitutes an enduring agenda within the oncology community. In a specialized research project under the leadership of Fetuma Feyera of the Department of Psychiatry at the Ambo University College of Medicine in Ethiopia the issues related to the depth and breadth of common mental disorders among cancer patients in Ethiopia as recorded in the Black Lion Specialized Hospital in Addis Ababa have been addressed (Feyera, Endeshaw, Kebede, Tirfessa, Bekele, 2022).

The uniqueness of this databased study and what makes it so significant and relevant to the on-going efforts globally to understand the range and nature of cancer care in developing societies is the focus upon the national hospital of Ethiopia in Addis Ababa, Ethiopia, Black Lion Specialized Hospital. Feyera and colleagues were aware of the generally recognized status of common mental disorders which frequently result from the patient's reaction to an initial cancer diagnosis resulting in emotional distress and psychological suffering. Though fully recognizing the need for databased evidence relevant to the nurturing of mental health and the development of professional intervention in a suffering patient's struggles with a cancer diagnosis, the team was quick to point out that very little hard data has been collected needed for Ethiopian medical professionals in their efforts to influence policy makers regarding the pressing need for reform in their national hospitals for the care of cancer patients facing the struggle with common mental disorders.

Focusing their attention upon the nationally distinguished treatment center at the Black Lion Specialized Hospital, the team directed their efforts primarily upon the assessment of the overwhelming magnitude of common mental disorders in Ethiopia including cognate factors present in cancer patients who experience a follow-up treatment at the Black Lion. Over a two month period in 2020, an institutional-based cross-sectional study was executed involving a systematic random sampling technique involving 396 cancer patients. Data was collected for this study employed a self-reporting questionnaire (SRQ-20) using an interviewer-administered structured questionnaire and the data was assessed based on a descriptive statistics and logistics regression model for analysis. In evaluating the response from 230 men and 160 women, there was an overall magnitude of common mental disorder among these cancer patients at a rate of 70% (73.5% for women and 67.8% for men) in the immediately preceding four weeks. Among the women with cancer suffering from a mental illness, these women were reported to be unemployed, averaging a monthly income below 1,600 Ethiopian Birr ($28.00 USA) and having been on cancer treatment over a 5 year time period with little or no social support and reliant upon substance abuse which led the researchers to identify these variables as significantly linked to common mental disorders.

The researchers recognized that common mental disorders are most prevalent among cancer patients and a significant characteristic of women in this study more so than among Ethiopian men particularly those using a psychoactive substance. The team concluded their study by suggesting that these cancer patients require particular attention from both the attending physicians as well as the mental health professionals specifically to be aware of any signs of mental distress or disorders which also provide an opportunity for social and economic services within the country to play a part in the care of this specialized group of cancer patients.

The care for a patient with a mental illness is challenging as is that of the care for a patient suffering from cancer. But when the patient is comorbid such that both a cancer diagnosis and a mental disorder is present, the life of both the patient and the patient's attending family and community support are profoundly affected. Studies of patient behavior and that of the medical team attending the patient are plentiful but fewer studies have actually focused upon the central importance of the family and social support. In light of the sparsity of databased and qualitative studies of this particular component of overall care of the cancer patient with a mental disorder, Kerri A. Murphy at the Massachusetts General Hospital and Harvard Medical School has put together a team of medical professionals specifically to address this deficient in research (Murphy, Corveleyn, Park, Irwin, et al., 2023). Their overall interest was the recognition and analysis of the challenges, rewards, as well as lessons to be learned from an examination of the personal accounts of family members and the network of community support individuals involved in the care of a cancer patient with a mental disorder.

Rather than an expansive databased study Murphy and team chose to use a qualitative interview method applied to 13 caregivers (9 family caregivers and 4 community caregivers) of patients diagnosed with head and neck, breast, lung, and gastrointestinal cancer suffering concurrently from a severe mental illness. The respondents agreed to participate in a single-arm pilot of person-centered collaborative care and were subjected to interviews which were transcribed and analyzed using both an inductive and inductive approach in response to the research team's specifically designed coding scheme based on the guidelines for the interviews which were double-coded and the topical themes within the context of a content analysis model. This approach also required a distinction in the interviewing process to be made between the two types of caregivers, viz., family and community.

Challenges faced in this approach to the topical theme of the research were substantial. They included the fundamental impact mental health symptoms face concerning the timing of the diagnosis, the treatment protocol, and the interplay between the care of the patient and the lack of resources linked particularly to the serious mental illness being faced by the patient receiving the care. An overriding interest and concern on the part of the family caregivers was reflected in the high valuation they placed on both closeness to the patient and the meaningfulness of that relationship. Both caregiver types, family and community, reported feeling a strong sense of efficacy in their role in this person-centered care model which they believed proved measurably beneficial to the patient under care. Beyond what the caregivers perceived to be the benefits of their working with the patient was the discovery that there were crucial lessons to be learned by themselves as well such as the central importance of attending to their own personal needs while in the service to the patient and the value of the role of advocate for the patient. They also reported that a team approach in this process resulted in the recognition of a devolution of mental health stigma felt often by the patient as well as perceived in the general public.

Acknowledging and validating the range of challenges as well as rewards experienced by the two types of caregivers in this study, viz., family and community, these researchers called for a more self-consciously driven design of approaches to be implemented in the care of cancer patients with severe mental illness reliant upon family and community caregiving support. More must be done in the area of research relative to both caregiver-patient linkage and non-spousal family caregivers if a better understanding of the role of informed intervention is to be embraced.

As commonly occurs within the general population, there is even within the health care community an unintended tendency to perceive a patient with a mental disability as somewhat less susceptible to health care such that there inevitably emerges a blatant disparity and inequality in the care and treatment of a cancer patient suffering from mental illness. Without intending to disparage the patient and not purposefully providing an inequitable quality of care, nevertheless, the perception of a cancer patient with mental illness is quite frequently the victim of a casual disregard for vigilance and robust health care practices on the part of the medical professionals responsible for patient care. Recognizing the need to maintain a high quality of care for all cancer patients, both the medical team and the psychiatric professionals working in tandem are called upon to present a high quality of conscientious care across the full spectrum of patients with comorbidities.

Cancer patients suffering from mental illness are particularly at risk of being viewed by the medical team as less likely to benefit from a vigorous attention to treatment protocols. Yuto Yamada of the Department of Neuropsychiatry at the Okayama University Graduate School in Japan was particular cognizant of the danger of slippage in quality care based on the medical attendants' perception of cancer patients diagnosed with psychiatric disorders. In response to this concern, Yamada put together a distinguished Japanese team of oncologists and medical professionals working with cancer patients with psychiatric issues for the specific purpose of delineating those factors which indicate misinformed perceptions with an eye towards offering corrective measures for their mitigation (Yamada, Fujiwara, Etho, Wada, et al., 2023). By focusing this research project on the psychiatric care providers' perceptions of cancer patients with mental illness, the aim was to reduce the blatant disparities between cancer patients without mental illness, who fair better in treatment care, and cancer patients with mental illness, who fair poorer in treatment care. The team is looking for factors and issues which are insufficiently addressed or prove to be difficult to identify on the part of the medical professionals tending to these cancer patients. Being fully cognizant of the difficulties involved in this type of performance and attitudinal care, this team was keen not to cast dispersions upon the health care team but to call attention to areas which might be improved in the care of cancer patients with mental illness thereby avoiding the disparities and inequities evident in clinical studies to-date.

Focusing on the Japanese health care system, the team surveyed psychiatric care providers at 23 psychiatric hospitals by means of a mail-in questionnaire. The questionnaire was based on four categories of information relevant to insufficiencies and difficulties in cancer care for the patient with mental illness using a five-point Likert scale. There were 15 items which the respondents were asked to rate of the four categories of questions and the research team then analyzed the percentage of respondents answering "insufficient/difficult" for each item. Psychiatric care providers responded at a 76.3% rate producing 255 completed responses of which questions relevant to both skills and attitudes of psychiatric professionals with above 50% responding that they sensed that attempts at promoting cancer screening and subsequent treatment were evaluated insufficient. Furthermore, items relative to collaborations between cancer and psychiatric care providers, just over 75% of the respondents felt that support for the cancer patient based on inpatient visitations involving the psychiatric and cancer hospital personnel were insufficient. Finally, questions related to in-psychiatric-hospital medical systems showed a variance of from 50% to 87% of the respondents assessing that support for screening, diagnosis/treatment, and palliative care for psychiatric inpatients proved insufficient/difficult with upwards of 42% to 57% evaluating the social services in the patient's community as insufficient.

The team set out to clarify the levels of insufficiency/difficulty recognized and assessed by the psychiatric care providers related to issues of significance to the care of cancer patients with mental illness. Within the health care community, psychiatric care providers are required to have been trained in the knowledge of and skills needed in cancer screening and treatment. They concluded that in order for there to be an improvement in cancer prevention, treatment, and palliative care, it is mandatory that developed systems of care to promote coordination between cancer hospitals and psychiatric hospitals must be addressed.

As with many if not all medically diagnosed conditions, the range of symptomatic presentations can be staggeringly complex and certainly with a cancer diagnosis due to the spectrum of cancer types and stages of development. So it is likewise with a diagnosis of a mental illness such that the types of mental illness range from mild anxiety to schizophrenia and the level of severity with each type of mental illness covers the spectrum of significance from mild to severe (aka serious). In order to assess the efficacy of cancer screening it must be linked to the level of commitment on the part of the patient to honor the treatment regimen set by the oncology team. This regimen is established on the basis of the type and severity of the cancer and linked to the type and severity of the patient's diagnosed mental illness. Measuring the efficacy of cancer screening required the team to identify the type of cancer and the stage of development at the time of screening and then to link it to the type and severity of mental illness experienced by the patient. Benedicte Kirkoen of the Cancer Registry of Norway has put together a team of oncology professionals from a range of institutions in Norway and the University of Glasgow in Scotland. The aim of this team's research effort was to more clearly understand the relevance of the participation of a patient diagnosed with colorectal cancer to the available screening protocol in relationship to that patient's type and severity of a diagnosed mental illness (Kirkoen, Berstad, Hoff, Bernkley, et al., 2023). Colorectal cancer is the number 2 cause of mortality globally.

The driving domain assumption validated by databased studies is that the overall effectiveness of colorectal cancer screening programs is specifically linked to the rate of participation. What interested this team of researchers was the link between the type and severity of mental illness to the participation of the patient in the screening program who has a diagnosis of colorectal cancer. If this methodological approach to this specific issue proves helpful, clearly the team was aware that it might be further applied to other types of cancer. The numerical scope of their database was impressive from the start from between 2012 and 2017, some 46,919 cancer patients were given the opportunity to participate in the sigmoidoscopy screening program in Norway as well as another 70,019 cancer patients were invited to participate in fecal immunochemical testing during the same time period. Subsequent to these test in 2022 the team used a logistic regression to actually evaluate the link between the use of antipsychotics, anxiolytics, hypnotics, and antidepressants immediately following the screening participation within the first year. Controlling for demographic and socioeconomic factors, the team tracked the daily doses of these specific drugs which were used to evaluate the dose-response relationship experienced by each participant.

Respondents who reported using at least one psychotropic medication was just short of 20% composite total with women showing 24.8% and men 13.4%. Furthermore, 60.7% of the non-participating patients screened used an anxiolytics and 64.3% used antipsychotics which increased over time in higher doses. The connection between hypnotics and antidepressants was evaluated as weak among nonparticipating patients using higher doses. The team was able to conclude from this databased study that there existed a significant disparity in colorectal cancer screening participation among patients diagnosed with a mental illness independent and distinct from the screening method used in this study. Furthermore, there was a registered variance in screening participation on the part of patients depending upon the type and severity of mental illness. These researchers called for targeted interventions for patients with a mental illness with emphasis upon the benefits of access to colorectal cancer screening.

CHAPTER TWO

Types of Cancer related to Mental Illness

Breast Cancer; Prostate Cancer; Lung Cancer; PTSD, Geriatric Cancer; Colorectal Cancer; Cervical Cancer; Laryngeal Cancer; Gynecologic Cancer; Schizophrenia

A special feature of oncology research is the range of specializations which are emerging throughout the world community. That lung cancer and breast cancer are two of the greatest killers have resulted in massive amounts of research and funding into these two types of cancer. However, other types of cancer have received a tremendous amount of databased studies in the past decades and combine that with an interest in the classification of cancer patients into age groups and a whole range of research opportunities become evident. To specialize in one type of cancer for a specific age group has become a common *modus operandi* for researchers and funding. Niranjan J. Sathianathen of the Department of Urology at the University of Minnesota in the USA has chosen to address a specific topic regarding the disparities of treatment among geriatric bladder cancer patients related to survival rates of such patients suffering from a pre-existing mental illness. Joined by several colleagues from the University of Minnesota, this team of researchers has identified a particularly overlooked group of cancer patients, namely, elderly bladder cancer patients with a mental illness linked to a measurable survival rate (Sathianathen, Fan, Jarosek, et al., 2020). The team centered their attention upon the statistically verified commonly known fact that geriatric patients with a pre-existing mental illness experience poor results from care and outcomes but no significant studies have focused upon bladder cancer specifically. This omission in research is addressed by this team of oncologists with special interest in the survival rates of the elderly.

Using the patient roster provided by the Surveillance, Epidemiology, and End Results (SEER)-Medicare database, this team conducted a retrospective analysis in which they identified elderly patients over the age of 68 years who suffered from a localized bladder cancer during the period of time from 2004 to 2011. This roster of patients was stratified based on pre-existing records of mental illness at the time cancer was diagnosed categorized as severe mental illness (including bipolar disorder, schizophrenia, and unspecified psychiatric disorders) anxiety, and depression. The team sought to compare the stages of presentation of cancer and receipt of guideline therapies such as radical cystectomy for muscle-invasive disease by employing a multivariable logistic regression analysis. Then, using the Kaplan-Meier analysis, they examined survival rates between these cancer patients who were suffering from a pre-existing mental disorder and those who did not have a diagnosed mental illness.

The database provided to the research team included 66,476 patient cases for analysis of which 4,468 had a recorded pre-existing mental disorder diagnosis at the time their cancer was diagnosed. Interestingly, these patients with previously diagnosed mental illness who developed bladder cancer were much more likely to manifest muscle-invasive disease than patients without an identified mental illness. The research team discovered that these patients with muscle-invasive disease who also suffered from a severe mental illness or depression actually were substantially less likely to submit to radical cystectomy or tri-modality therapy. However, of those patients who actually did undergo radical cystectomy manifested substantially superior overall survival results as compared to patients who did not undergo these curative treatment measures.

What proved most disturbing to the research team was the fact that guideline-concordant management was much less likely to be offered to geriatric patients suffering from muscle-invasive bladder cancer with a diagnosed mental disorder which clearly was responsible for a decline in the overall quality of care and survival. Research showed that these cancer patients who were concurrently suffering from severe mental illness and depression were significantly disinclined to receive radical cystectomy for muscle-invasive disease and thus were not able to take advantage of guideline-concordant treatment. Survival rates were, of course, significantly lower in patients which pre-existing mental illness and where disease-specific survival was understandably lower for those patients not receiving guideline-concordant care.

Oncological research and medical practice have accelerated over the past few decades such that specializations have proliferated throughout the medical world in the form of research programs, specialized institutions, advanced post-credential training, and particularly in the form of scholarly publications. The literature is replete with specializations within cancer research and all of this refinement has led to a deepening of medical science's understanding of the complexities and range of cancer types which now call for focused attention. Bladder cancer has received a monumental amount of funded research in the areas of particularly physical prognostic assessments involving nutritional and performance such that the on-going development of research data now indicates that both pre- and post-treatment of mental health, a new focus of interest, may significantly impact the patient's long-term well-being reflected in the patient's physical health. Hannah Phan, a urological oncologist from the Texas Tech University Health Sciences Centers has been joined by two research colleagues from the same health system to make a formal inquiry into the impact upon mental health a bladder cancer diagnosis may have (Pham, Torres, Sharma, 2019). Beyond concerns in oncological care of the bladder patient regarding nutrition, performance, and physical state at the time of diagnosis and follow-through, this team was particularly focused upon the psychosocial spectrum of bladder cancer care such that not just the bio-medical but the psychosocial aspects of patient care must be factored into the health care protocol.

In their attempt to sort out and delineate factors resulting from diagnostic and treatment protocols for patients with bladder cancer as having an impact upon the mental health of the patient, Pham and colleagues did a comprehensive review of literature dealing with the subject. Exploring a standard industry-wide approved approach to literature review and summarization, they conducted a modified, non\systematic analysis covering the years 2000 to 2018 as found in PubMed, Web of Science, EMBASE, SCOPUS, and OVID sources. They focused upon a few carefully selected terms and concepts restricted to English-language, peer-reviewed, original research, viz., *bladder cancer, non-muscle-invasive bladder cancer, muscle-invasive bladder cancer, mental health, psychological distress, depression, and suicide.* The research team scanned 87 publications falling into this category and selected 19 articles which proved relevant specifically to the topic at hand. Each of the key terms and concepts were identified within the relevant periodical such that each term and concept was covered in the published literature.

As in the case of cancer and suicide explored in my previous book (Morgan, 2023b) *Cancer and Suicide: A Resource Compendium of Published Research,* there is a disturbingly high rate of cancer patients suffering from a full range of mental illnesses. As we have shown in the case of the global reality of the high prevalence of the cancer and suicide matrix, so with cancer and mental illness which shows no bias with respect to nationality and an expansive spectrum of converging variables not least of which is that of the presence of mental illness among patients with breast cancer. Alex J. Mitchell of the Department of Psycho-oncology at the University of Leicester in the UK and his colleagues set about to address the meagerness of data related to prevalence of mental illness among breast cancer patients in a 2014 study (Mitchell, et al., 2014). Of particular interest to Mitchell and his research team was that of the specifically identified linkage, if such really exists, between breast cancer patients and a designated rate of mental illness. They used a comparative meta-analysis of mammography uptake with special attention to the question as to whether or not women with identified mental health issues are more or less likely to access mammography screening compared to women designated mentally healthy.

Using a commonly employed mammography screening instrument based on odds ratios linked to a randomized meta-analysis identifying women with and without mental illness, the findings were subsequently stratified using a common primary diagnosis consisting of any identified mental illness such as mood disorders, depression, severe mental illness, distress and anxiety. Basing their statistical analysis drawn from 24 scholarly publications in the field reporting breast cancer screening results of some 715,705 women with mental illness and drawing further data from 5 additional studies screening 21,491 women experiencing distress but not demonstrating mental disorder symptoms, they found that in pooling the data from this meta-analysis there proved to be a significantly measurable reduction in the rates of mammography screening in women with identified mental illness, mood disorders, and especially severe mental illness. Interestingly enough, there was no measurable disparity among women suffering from distress only. Clearly from the data, women with mental illness are much less likely to undergo mammography screening and this is particularly true of women suffering from severe mental illness. A red flag of caution and awareness had to do with evidence showing that the presence of emotional distress is linked to disparities in medical care due to mental illness in the patient and this calls for a redress within the treatment field of oncology.

Medical research has shown a consistent pattern among women with serious mental illness (SMI) who also suffer from cervical and breast cancer with a strong tendency to decline screening such that in the failure of the uptake there is a lack of data regarding screening factors of identification and treatment as well as avoidance of primary care consultation. The correlation between a lapse in the uptake of women with cancer and serious mental illness constitutes a significant field of pressing databased research. Charlotte Woodhead of the Institute of Psychiatry, Psychology and Neuroscience at King's College, London was joined by several of her colleagues in various departments at the College along with a member of the University of Otago in Wellington, NZ, in an attempt to fill the void in this field of research (Woodhead, Cunningham, et al., 2016).

The level of research methodological sophistication was enhanced by the research team in using logistic regression models which were adjusted for both socio-demographic factors as well as for primary care consultation frequency. By linking both population-based primary and secondary care data taken from a borough in London (UK), the team was able to compare breast and cervical cancer screening receipts for both patients suffering from serious mental illness (n=625 and n=1,393 respectively) with patients who were not suffering from a serious mental illness identified only by primary care records (n=106,554 and =25,385 respectively).

Of relevance to interest in uptake data relative to the subjects being analyzed, i.e., women suffering from serious mental illness suffering from breast and cervical cancer, they found that these SMI patients were commonly provided with breast and cervical screening. They did find that patients diagnosed with schizophrenia, antipsychotic prescriptions, illness severity and risk of mental illness were clearly linked to the lowest rate of uptake breast and cervical screening. A further exacerbating factor leading to a reduction in effectiveness for the SMI patient was linked to consultation frequency for cervical screening.

An anticipated finding in this research was that women suffering from a serious mental illness are commonly less likely to seek or receive breast and cervical cancer screening as opposed to women suffering from such cancer but without diagnosable SMI. The team concluded that an increase in the primary care rate of consultation among SMI patients should constitute a mediating factor between this classification of patient and the uptake especially for cervical screening customarily available through formal primary care protocols. The key, they suggested to improving and elevating screening uptake among this classification of patients suffering from disparities result most frequently from SMI. However, this may also improve overall care of women with other illnesses and those at risk of such not just limited to SMI patients.

Certain types of cancer at all stages of diagnosis and development have enjoyed the lion's share of research funding and interest over the past 50 years. As is self-evident, breast cancer tops this list of favorite topics within the oncology community. What has until recent decades received less attention is breast cancer patients suffering from a morbidity of mental illness and psychiatric disorders. Early on in cancer research history, there was the recognition that cancer and mental illness often constitute a companionable pair of medical issues but research addressing specifically breast cancer and mental illness has received less attention. Kristy Iglay of the Rutgers School of Public Health in New Jersey has chosen to pinpoint this void in research by calling upon colleagues from the Rutgers School as well as researchers in the Rutgers Cancer Institute of New Jersey and the Rutgers Robert Wood Johnson Medical School. The specific focus of this team's research was upon the diagnosis and treatment of elderly breast cancer patients suffering from mental illness (Iglay, Santorelli, Hirshfield, et al., 2017). The particular point of research interest had to do with the variance between elderly breast cancer patients with mental illness versus those without an identified mental disorder with a specific interest in focusing upon diagnosis and treatment protocols.

From the earliest days the challenge to oncologists working with psychiatric disorders and mental illness in cancer patients, the classification of the various types of mental illness has necessarily been relegated to the categorical identifications established by the International Classification of Diseases (ICD) as reported in the Ninth Revision Clinical Modification codes. This recognized authority in mental illness identification as used by the research team during the 3 year period prior to the study group's cancer diagnosed patients, both in and out of hospital, as either having no mental illness or suffering from a range of disorders such as anxiety, depression, and severe mental illness including bipolar disorder, schizophrenia, and other unspecified psychotic disorders. The team used the data provided by the Surveillance, Epidemiology and End Results-Medicare (SEER) resources covering 16,636 women 68 years of age and older who had been diagnosed with breast cancer ranging from stage I to stage IIIa in the U..S. for the years 2005 to 2007.

As has been consistently pointed out through this investigation of published research in the past decade, certain types of cancer at all stages of diagnosis and development have enjoyed the lion's share of research funding and interest over the past 50 years. Breast cancer tops this list of favorite research topics within the oncology community. What has until recent decades received less attention is breast cancer patients suffering from a morbidity of mental illness and psychiatric disorders. Early on there was the recognition that cancer and mental illness often constitute a companionable pair of medical issues but research addressing specifically breast cancer and mental illness has received less attention. Kristy Iglay of the Rutgers School of Public Health in New Jersey has chosen to pinpoint this void in research by calling upon colleagues from the Rutgers School as well as researchers in the Rutgers Cancer Institute of New Jersey and the Rutgers Robert Wood Johnson Medical School. Published in the *Journal of Clinical Oncology* in December following the November research paper published in thc *Breast Cancer Research Treatment* journal, the specific focus of this team's research was upon the diagnosis and treatment of elderly breast cancer patients suffering from mental illness (Iglay, Santorelli, Hirshfield, et al., 2017). The particular point of research interest had to do with the variant results between elderly breast cancer patients with mental illness versus those without an identified mental disorder focusing upon diagnosis and treatment protocols.

As has been consistently the challenge to oncologists working with psychiatric disorders and mental illness in cancer patients, the classification of the various types of mental illness has necessarily been relegated to the categorical identifications established by the International Classification of Diseases as reported in the Ninth Revision Clinical Modification codes. This recognized authority in mental illness identification as used by the research team during the 3 year period prior to the study group's cancer diagnosis designated patients, both in and out of hospital, as either having no mental illness or suffering from a range of disorders such as anxiety, depression, and severe mental illness including bipolar disorder, schizophrenia, and other unspecified psychotic disorders. The team used the data provided by the Surveillance, Epidemiology and End Results-Medicare resources covering 16,636 women 68 years of age and older who had been diagnosed with breast cancer ranging from stage I to stage IIIa in the U..S. for the years 2005 to 2007.

A regularly exasperating situation for oncologists is whether or not and to what extent there is a barrier to cancer patients, and in this study particularly hereditary breast cancer and ovarian cancer patients (HBOC), to seek out and submit to genetic counseling relative to the patient's medical situation. A further complicating variable is related to the ethnicity of the patient and the legal and ethical issues involved in patient identification has constituted a monumentally important matrix of concerns experienced by the research team of Marra G. Ackerman of the Langone Medical Center of New York University along with colleagues from the Columbia University Medical Center in New York City (Ackerman, Shapiro, Coe, Trivedi, Crew, 2017). The driving force in this research project was to what extent and the nature of the impact mental illness had upon the uptake of genetic counseling for HBOC patients drawn from a multiethnic cohort of patients suffering from breast cancer.

Selecting 308 women with newly diagnosed breast cancer from academic urban medical centers in the New York Cityarea from the years 2007 to 2015 who qualified for the HBOC genetic testing program, the team conducted a retrospective analysis of this cohort relative to an uptake of genetic services including a personal history of mental health disorders (MHD). These were characterized as constituting a psychiatric diagnosis and/or treatment of patients with antidepressant, mood stabilizer, anxiolytic, or antipsychotic medications. This information was accessed through medical chart reviews with the mean age of women with breast cancer diagnosed at 56 years broken down into ethnic groups of non-Hispanic whites at 44%, Hispanics at 37%, and non-Hispanic Blacks at 15th. Of this total cohort, 32% (n=99) women qualified for the MHD designation with 73% having a genetic referral, 57% having undergone genetic counseling with 54% actually having completed the BRCA testing which looks for

DNA changes that increase the risk of breast cancer and ovarian cancer. Though the research team learned that the uptake of genetic counseling services did not vary significantly by race and ethnicity or by presence of mental health issues, they did discover that in a multivariable analysis, younger patients of Ashkenazi Jewish heritage and a family history of breast cancer were clearly linked with HBOC genetic counseling. What was evident to the research team was that a significant percentage of patients suffering from breast cancer proved to qualify for HBOC genetic testing resulting in a referral to genetic counseling, noting that these referrals did not vary according to mental health issues or race and ethnicity designations.

A perpetual challenge to oncologists is the disparity between what is medically known about cancer and the ability of the patient to grasp the overall assessment and treatment of that cancer given the fact that most patients have no medical training to actually understand the complexities of the diagnosis, prognosis, or treatment protocols. This reality is further complicated exponentially with cancer patients who have a history of psychiatric disorders and mental illness such as schizophrenia, dementia, and intellectual disability. The enduring research question has to do with whether or not and/or to what extent this disparity between a cancer patient's understanding of the diagnosis who has a mental disorder versus the cancer patient who does not suffer from mental illness. Yoshiaki Shinden and a team of colleagues at the University Graduate School of Medical Sciences at Kagoshima, Japan, put together a carefully executed research tool designed to speak specifically to the clinical characteristics of breast cancer patients who were suffering from a mental disorder, particularly schizophrenia, dementia, and intellectual deficiencies (Shinden, Kijima, Hirata, Nakajo, et al., 2017).

It is commonly recognized within the diagnostic functions of the oncological team that severe mental illness can have a measurable impact upon the thoroughness of the diagnosis and the sophistication of the treatment for breast cancer patients in light of the frequently lower awareness of the cancer diagnosed and a general understanding of cancer itself. This void or deficiency in the patient's understanding of the situation inevitably and understandably reduces the medical team's ability to rely upon a congenial and cooperative spirit within the patient. This team, therefore, set out to analyze the multitude of clinical characteristics of breast cancer patients who suffered from pre-existing mental disorders such as schizophrenia, dementia, and intellectual disability or deficiency. The sample of 46 patients who had a diagnosis of schizophrenia, dementia, or intellectual disability but prior to a breast cancer diagnosis constituted the basis for this research. This group was compared with a control group of 727 breast cancer patients who did not have a diagnosed mental disorder during the study (3 patients actually had more than 2 mental disorders as diagnosed by the psychiatric staff). All participants of the study group underwent a curative surgical treatment for breast cancer between September of 1992 and January of 2015. The findings of this study group with clinico-pathological data was compared to the 727 control group patients.

Due partially to the intellectual disability of the study group members, some of the patients with mental disorders were actually not cognizant of their own breast cancer lesions such that the cancer was often identified by family members or health care workers and not infrequently by the medical team itself. Patients identified as having mental disorders actually registered a significantly higher rate of advanced T factors (size factor) and overall stage of cancer development at the time of surgery than patients who did not manifest diagnosable mental illness. However, more patients underwent total mastectomy but fewer patients underwent postoperative adjuvant chemotherapy and radiation. Two fundamentally insightful findings which were not expected was the fact that biological markers such as estrogen receptors, progesterone receptors, and human epidermal growth factors were not significantly different between breast cancer patients with mental disorders and those without. Furthermore and finally, the research team discovered that the outcomes for patients with mental disorders were not worse than for those patients without mental disorders. This discovery necessarily precipitated a call for more detailed and advanced research on the differentiation between breast cancer patients with mental disorders and those without.

In order to avoid the disastrous pitfalls of a biased moralizing regarding the medical treatment of patients generally and in this study of cancer patients with mental illness particularly, it does rest with the research community in oncological studies to account for often blatant disparities of treatment when variables such as comorbidity and mental illness are factored into the rate of mortality. Any attempt at an explanatory justification for bold disparities when identifying variables characterizing a category of cancer patients treads too closely to the line of poor assessment or quality of care in the absence of statistical clarification when elevated mortality rates for certain categories of cancer patients is in question. Aulikki J. Ahlgren-Rimpilainen of the National Institute for Health and Welfare in Helsinki (Finland) has drawn public attention to the reality of such disparities when dealing specifically with women with breast cancer suffering from a severe mental illness. Joined by a panel of distinguished Finnish medical researchers from the Helsinki medical community, Ahlgren-

Rimpilainen initiated a comprehensive study of this issue in Finland drawing from data provided by the Finnish Cancer Registry and from the Hospital Discharge Register (Ahlgren-Rimpilainen, Arffman, Suvisaari, et al., 2020).

Beginning with the indisputable statement that women with breast cancer suffering from severe mental illness (SMI) have a documented elevated level of mortality. The disparity between breast cancer patients with mental illness and those without mental illness, this disparity has not been systematically studied in terms of differential rates of treatment survival and mortality. This Finnish team from the staff of the National Institute for Health and Welfare in Helsinki set out to address this information gap in the understanding of this blatant disparity in treatment. Three factors were considered in comparing breast cancer specific mortality with those patients who suffered from a severe mental illness and those who did not. They focused research on the treatment impact affecting the stage of cancer at initial presentation, comorbidity, and actual differences in treatment protocols.

Using the Finnish Cancer Registry, some 80,671 women with their first breast cancer diagnosis were identified with 4,837 women listing their previous hospital admissions as reported by the Hospital Discharge Register. Finally, records for the causes of death statistics were also considered in this analysis with the team employing competing risk models. There was a recorded significant elevation in breast cancer mortality for women with severe mental illness when the analysis controlled for age, the year of cancer diagnosis, and actual comorbidity. Though their records reported a somewhat higher mortality rate for breast cancer patients manifesting no affective psychosis, the team made the suggestion that a viable explanation could be the relevance of the patient's reported stage of cancer presentation. Furthermore the research showed that both substance use and mood disorders contributed to a substantial increase in mortality among women with breast cancer.

Finally and tellingly insightful was the statistical verification that breast cancer patients suffering from a severe mental illness actually received much less radiotherapy than patients not suffering from a psychiatric disorder. The team concluded this monumentally important study by calling for an improvement in early detection of breast cancer of women suffering from severe mental illness, emphasizing the importance of collegial consultation between mental health workers and oncologists.

A companioned agenda for research oncology is to both explore the long-term benefits of newly developed cancer care treatments and protocols and also to track the efficacy over time of already established methods of cancer care covering a full range of patients. One of the key watchwords in this field is that of disparities and inequities in the treatment of a full spectrum of cancer types and cancer patients assessed on the basis of the psychosocial factors characterizing each patient. To complicate the tracking of such issues is the introduction of severe mental illness into the diagnostic matrix such that not only do researchers wish to know all that can be known at this time about a specific type of cancer and the patients it infects but also to what extent any and all cancer assessment, diagnosis, and treatment protocols are affected when the patient has a pre-existing severe mental illness or psychiatric disorder. This last issue has not always been either recognized or a concern for oncology research which historically has focused upon the biochemical and molecular characteristics of the various types of cancer. In recent years, the research spectrum has been broadened by the development of psychiatric oncology which addresses issues related to the psychosocial spectrum of cancer care including the presence of severe mental illness in the patient.

A growing area of special concern addressing the issues characterizing the disparities and inequities of cancer treatment is that of the central importance of a diagnosis of a severe mental illness preceding the cancer. Steve Kisely of the University of Queensland's School of Clinical Medicine in Australia has put together a research team of oncologists and psychiatrists focused specifically upon the nature of these disparities characterizing the quality of breast cancer treatment of patients suffering from mental illness (Kisely, Alotiby, Protani, Soole, 2023). The concern in the research agenda is that of the mortality rate of breast cancer patients with a pre-existing severe mental illness (SMI) including particularly schizophrenia, bipolar disorder, and major depression. The death rate among these specific patients is somewhat higher than that of the general public. The initial surmise was that the infrequent cancer screening among cancer patients with a mental disorder might account for some of the measured disparities but in the absence of hard data to validate this surmise coupled with the possibility of other unidentified barriers to quality and regular treatment following diagnosis must not be overlooked.

The first step to investigate these apparent disparities was to begin with a systematic review and meta-analysis of the issue related to the guidelines accessible for appropriate treatment subsequent to a breast cancer diagnosis. Particular attention to these specific patients who were suffering from a severe mental illness prior to the cancer diagnosis was of primary concern. This included patients who were the recipients of cancer treatments such as surgery, endocrine, and chemo- or radiotherapy. In pursuit of a substantial database of patients under breast cancer treatment both with a pre-existing SMI and those without, the team searched for indexed articles listed in these key resources, i.e., PubMed, EMBASEW, PsychInfo, and CINAHL. Population-based cohorts and case-control studies were of particular relevance to this databased research agenda. Following the identification of some 13 relevant studies in this review of literature, the team determined that there were 4 studies which actually proved relevant with adjusted outcomes to the meta-analysis undertaken by the team. A disturbing find in this databased study was that patients suffering from a severe mental illness were less likely to secure guideline-appropriate care and these same patients had a longer time to wait to receive appropriate care when finally available. Mixed results occurred even with an unadjusted assessment of these SMI patients for such variables as age, comorbidities, and stage of cancer diagnosis for such factors as surgery, hormone, radio- or chemotherapy.

This team found conclusive databased evidence that breast cancer patients suffering from a severe mental illness actually received either less or significantly delayed guideline-appropriate care for their breast cancer than members of the general public. These researchers suggested that further study of these disparities is called for given their findings in which mortality rates were substantially higher among breast cancer patients suffering from a severe mental illness due to a failure of accessibility and quality of care when offered.

As is common with most serious illnesses, there is always the possibility of there being other health issues complicating the diagnosis of a specific illness such that a carefully constructed awareness of and response to the comorbidity conditions present in the patient usually proves of great benefit in a proper and comprehensive assessment and treatment of the whole person. As is commonly known in oncology, a cancer diagnosis almost always carries with it either the danger of inducing an emotional stress situation or, not so uncommon, the discovery of a pre-existing mental illness at the time of the cancer diagnosis. In addition, recognition of comorbidity possibilities is crucial. Not only is it crucial for there to be the identification of other health issues in a patient diagnosed with cancer but also equally important is the identification of the types of health issues characterizing the cancer patient's overall physical status. Comorbidity status is fundamental in understanding the relationship of a mental disorder in patients suffering from cancer in order to more fully assess the patient's overall health. Huah Shin Ng of the College of Medicine and Public Health at Flinders University in Adelaide, Australia has put together a research agenda focusing precisely on this matrix of health issues involving cancer patients with a mental illness and the comorbidities which might be present in the patient at the time of diagnosis (Ng, Woodman, Koczwara, 2023).

In spite of the recognition within the medical community of the relevance of comorbidities when diagnosing a patient and establishing a treatment protocol, there is still a limited number of databased studies addressing specifically the relevance of a comorbidity awareness when dealing with a cancer patient suffering from a mental illness or psychiatric disorder. Though the seeming self-evidence of the impact that comorbidity will have upon a cancer diagnosis when complicated by a concurrent mental illness, there is still a sparsity of research delineating specifically those factors which might prove beneficial in a comprehensive health care plan for a cancer patient in this situation. Ng and colleagues from the College of Medicine at Flinders University set about to address this research weakness in a databased analysis by launching a cross-sectional analysis based on data made available from the Australian National Health Survey (2017-2018) consisting of all respondents over the age of 25 years who either had a history of cancer or did not. Individual and cluster comorbidities in this study group were measured against the poor health and mental distress based on the respondent's cancer status.

From the national data base made available to this research team, there were 1,982 patients with cancer (52% female) and 12,635 without cancer (51% female). Patients who reported having cancer were commonly older and subject to a comorbidity as opposed to the younger non-cancer patients. With the exceptions of skin conditions and infectious diseases, these older respondents were commonly in poorer health than those non-cancer patients for each reported comorbidity. And, with the adjusted odds ratio for digestive disorders and blood conditions, the most evident linkage with poor health and mental distress manifested itself most often in patients with a comorbid mental illness. What proved helpful in this analysis was an exploratory cluster analysis which identified four specific comorbidity clusters including low comorbidity, musculoskeletal, respiratory and cardio-metabolic. The research showed that cancer survivors in the cardio-metabolic cluster actually had a higher reported rate of poor health as well as mental distress than patients with a lower rate of comorbidity. What the team found conclusively was that cancer survivors with comorbidities was a common phenomenon and this was linked to a poorer health status the severity of which was dependent upon the specific type of comorbidity from which the patient suffered. The research team's suggestion to the health care community was that risk assessments and management of comorbidities should always constitute a significant point of priority in the care and treatment of cancer patients and cognate research.

As is well documented breast cancer among women constitutes a major field of research due to the pervasive nature of this disease. A complication to the oncological study of breast cancer among women is that of a pre-existing mental illness and a furtherance of this troubling illness among breast cancer patients is that of the age factor. Older women with breast cancer suffering from a mental illness comprise one of the great challenges in diagnosis and treatment protocols due more precisely to the nature of a psychiatric disorder among these older patients. To research this composite of breast cancer, mental illness, and older age constitutes a significant constellation of variables worthy of closer scrutiny than may have been given in the past. This focus precipitated Manami Bhattacharya at the National Cancer Institute in Maryland to put together a research team from the University of Minnesota School of Public Health to launch a robust databased assessment of this tripartite constellation with the goal of delineating the profound impact that breast cancer and mental illness has upon older women in the U.S. (Bhattacharya, Parsons, Call, Blaes, McAlpine, 2023).

The research team began with the stated recognition that the presence of mental illness among women suffering from breast cancer constitutes an elevated risk of mortality with the knowledge that barriers to accessing cancer screening protocols and other recommended treatment programs may be to blame. The fact that the early detection of a cancer is a very important factor in breast cancer survival and, therefore, the team set out to delineate the factors affecting the disparity in survival rates among older women with breast cancer suffering from a mental illness. The overarching question posed by the research team was whether or not and to what extent older women with a diagnosed mental illness are fundamentally more susceptible to a diagnosis when there is a late-staged breast cancer as opposed to such women who have not been diagnosed with a mental illness. This is the enduring point of investigation.

The research plan developed by this team of medical professionals was thorough in every stage of development beginning with the SEER-Medicare data for 2005-2015 for the purpose of identifying AJCC stage I-IV breast cancer patients who either had or did not have a history of mental illness before their cancer diagnosis. The linkage between mental illness diagnoses and the cancer stage at diagnosis was based on the use of a generalized ordinal regression controlling for age, race/ethnicity, income, comorbidities, primary care use, rurality, and marital status. The delineation of the cohort totals was based on 96,034 women suffering from breast cancer and the percentage breakdown showed that 1.7% of the total had experienced a serious mental illness, 19.9% had suffered from depression or anxiety, and another 7.0% from other mental illnesses unspecified. What proved most informative was that 40% higher odds of being diagnosed with AJCC Stages II and III rather than Stage I characterized women with a serious mental illness. Women suffering from depression and anxiety showed a 25% lower odds rate of being diagnosed with Stage IV cancer rather than those with a Stage I diagnosis which was matched more or less by when suffering from other types of mental illnesses.

The researchers found that a higher mortality rate following breast cancer characterized women who had suffered from a serious mental illness but were, alas, diagnosed at later stages of cancer but women diagnosed with depression and anxiety actually demonstrated a lower risk of Stage IV cancer. The research team emphasized that breast cancer diagnoses earlier in women with a serious mental illness may prove to be an important goal for reducing the obvious disparities affecting breast cancer survival rates among this cohort of women patients.

Nationally-based, population-specific, and cancer typology databased studies constitute the most important concentration of research variables in understanding the nature of cancer within the human population. Karen M. Tuesley of the University of Queensland's school of public health in Herston, Australia, has been joined by research colleagues from Australian universities and health service institutes along with a colleague from the Dalhousie University in Canada to focus precisely upon these three components of cancer research (Tuesley, Jordan, Siskind, Kendall, Kisely, 2019). Concentrating their studies of Australians on the government's national health plan, Tuesley's research team selected the three most common types of cancer, i.e., colorectal, cervical, and prostate, to do a study of the function and effectiveness of the screening of these types of cancer patients who are suffering from severe mental illness (SMI). This retrospective nation-wide cohort study constituted the first major such study of its kind in Australia and it distinguished itself for addressing all three features, i.e., nationality, population specific, and cancer types in one monumental national study.

Granted that a measurably higher rate of mortality than in the general population exists among cancer patients suffering from severe mental illness, the team purposefully drew attention to the ambiguity of study results when measuring cancer screening among SMI patients and mortality rates of the same cohort. They chose to analyze the occurrence of these three types of cancer screening, viz., colorectal, cervical, and prostate, and the differences between these cancer patients in each of the three cohort groupings who were either suffering from SMI or not in the general Australian population among those participating in the national health care program of the government. The research team employed the Poisson regression in their efforts to anticipate incidence ratio rates based on a 95% confidence rate addressing the linkage between severe mental illness (SMI) and the measurable rates determined for fecal occult blood testing, pap smears, and prostate-specific antigen tests.

What the team found was that patients suffering from a severe mental illness (SMI) were actually linked to a 17% reduction rate of patients having a pap smear as well as patients who underwent a prostate-specific antigen test as compared to the general Australian population. However and on the other hand, they found that measurable rates of fecal occult blood testing proved to be actually lower among members of the cohort with severe mental illness who visited their own family physician no more than four times annually. The research team registered a concern that owing to a mismatching of data for cancer and rate of mortality in patients with severe mental illness, there is a strong possibility of a conflict in readings for the screening frequency among such patients. Therefore, they concluded that more care must be exercised in the improvement of preventive screening measures particularly among disadvantaged groups.

It is generally understood that the responsibility of psychiatric oncology is to address the psychosocial spectrum of cancer care as a manifestation of its specific domain of jurisdiction within the broad field of cancer care among oncologists. There is the realization on the part of psychiatric oncologists that patients suffering from prostate cancer are most susceptible to long-term issues of mental illness relative to that form of cancer as the duration of the treatment protocols extend often far beyond the timeframe of other forms of cancer treatment. To address the psychological issues implied in a prostate cancer diagnosis and in anticipation of mental illness issues arising from such constitutes a major focus of research interfacing personality traits and urinary symptoms which are commonly linked in a mental health distress matrix of prostate cancer patients. Charles Gillis of the Department of Urology at Dalhousie University in Halifax, Canada, has been joined by colleagues in cognate departments of epidemiology and radiation oncology at that university with the goal of explicating the factors affecting the mortality rate of prostate cancer patients with personality issues manifesting mental health distress in response to a diagnosis of prostate cancer. The interest in this specialized research agenda grew out of the awareness that prostate cancer patients often have a higher rate of mental illness arising from the cancer diagnosis which commonly lasts longer than in other forms of cancer. Since less research attention has been directed to this particular behavioral matrix, the Gillis team mobilized their research interest focused in the Canadian Maritime provinces (Gillis, Ilie, Mason, Bailly, et al., 2021).

Between May of 2017 and December of 2019, 189 men identified from the Canadian Maritime Provinces suffering from prostate cancer agreed to participate in a quality-of-life online survey dealing with cancer and mental illness. Differentiating between participants who had experienced screening for mental illness constituted the driving principle of this study. The team used the Kessler's 10-item scale (K10) and urinary symptoms in this study and also used the International Prostate symptom Score (IPSS). The ten-item personality inventory test (TIPI) was used to assess extraversion, agreeableness, conscientiousness, emotional stability (aka neuroticism), and an openness to new experiences. In order to assess the efficacy of the linkage between personality, urinary symptoms, and mental distress, the team developed a multivariate logistic regression model while controlling for time factors including time of diagnosis, treatment types, age of participants, and multi-morbidity of each patient.

The team was surprised to discover from the data analysis that there was no identifiable linkage between cancer treatment received by the patients for prostate cancer and personality types. However, they did find that screening positive for mental illness involved 18% of the participants in which there was a linkage between personality traits of low levels of emotional stability and moderate to severe urinary problems. Based on their data analysis, the team suggested in this study that screening for mental illness among patients with prostate cancer might see a reduction in morbidity linked to actual cancer treatment while identifying patients susceptibly at risk for mental health distress. They proposed that these patients may very well benefit from an individualized mental health support mechanism mobilized by both the oncology treatment staff as well as the sponsoring medical institution.

The diversity of research opportunities is illustrated by the proliferation of types of cancer which the American Society of Clinical Oncology lists at over 120 identifiably distinctive types. Some of these are extremely rare, such as Adrenal cortex carcinoma, while others constitute the most common types including lung, breast, prostate, and colorectal cancer. Though much progress is being made in the study and treatment of rare types of cancer, a lion's share of research and specializations within oncology are focused upon the four most common types with the realization that it is lung cancer which leads the mortality rate in the U.S. covering all spectra of races and ethnicities. One of the most beneficial addresses to the pervasive presence of lung cancer in the U.S. is that of cancer screening and particularly of cancer patients suffering from a serious mental illness. To that end, Efren J. Flores, Elyse R. Park, and Kelly E. Irwin of Massachusetts General Hospital and the Harvard Medical School have chosen to explore the various types of treatments used in the identification and diagnostic assessments of lung cancer relative to the significance of cancer screening particularly of serious mentally ill patients (Flores, Park, Irwin, 2019).

In spite of the fact that lung cancer is still the leading cause of cancer death in the United States across a spectrum of variables including ethnicity and age, there is the research realization that not all groups are equally affected and this is particularly true among lung cancer patients who have been diagnosed with a psychiatric disorder or mental illness. Research has shown that there is up to a 400% higher frequency rate of lung cancer among patients suffering from schizophrenia and bipolar disorder somewhat attributed to a higher rate of smoking addiction evidence in the general cancer population. This research shows it is commonly due to a patient's reluctance to seek a diagnosis or to choose to delay treatment which itself often proves inadequate or inequitable in various levels of conscientious care. Furthermore and continually exacerbating assessment, diagnosis, and treatment is the fact that lung cancer patients suffering from a serious mental illness are frequently confronted with systemic barriers to access cancer screening including such factors as cognitive deficiencies wherein the patient has little capacity to understand the nature and value of such screening. These cognitive encumbrances are not infrequently linked to poverty and social isolation, patient-provider relationship failures, reluctance to reduce tobacco attachments, and the inefficiency of much of primary care and mental health assessment and treatment. A surprising statistic validated by these researchers is that over against all of the publicly provided information regarding the benefits of cancer screening, the actual utilization of this cancer treatment service continues to fall below 4% of the national population annually. Even more disturbing is the team's observation that in recognition of the disparities among cancer screening accessibility and utilization by patients, they are convinced that the utilization rate among lung cancer patients suffering from a diagnosed serious mental illness is even lower. In conclusion, the team was hopeful that a pilot collaboration utilized between radiological oncology and psychiatric oncology carried with it a promise of significant benefits for lung cancer patients with serious mental illness who access available screening.

An enduring topic of research interest is that of the relationship between severe mental illness (SMI) and lung cancer mortality and this topic constitutes an internationally representative interest across ethnicities, genders, and nationalities. What often proves the most helpful in the actual practice of oncology is for the research to be geographically specific such that the data gathered and analyzed from a single country can constitute a potential contribution to the overall cancer care system in that country. Transnational studies have always been of benefit but Martti Arffman of the National Institute for Health and Welfare in Helsinki, Finland, has been joined by a team of oncological researchers in that country from major research universities to focus upon the current state of mental illness and lung cancer in Finland covering a 33 year period from 1990 to 2013. Arffman was joined by seven other specialists in this research project focusing upon the impact SMI has upon lung cancer mortality drawing data from a register-based cohort study (Arffman, Manderbacka, Suvisaari, et al., 2019). Arffman and team were fully aware of the internationally validated link between severe mental illness and its impact upon the elevation of cancer mortality but they were eager in this study to point out that though many internationally-based studies have consistently failed to address the topic of most interest to Arffman and team, namely, the relationship between SMI and lung cancer survival rates.

A unique feature of this study was that of comparing issues related to cancer-specific mortality in lung cancer patients for those who had a history of SMI as well as those who did not. The team analyzed the mortality rates and attempted to identify differences on the basis of the stages of cancer at the time of presentation, comorbidity and even differences in the cancer treatments used on each patient. Using the Finnish Cancer Registry, the team was able to locate patients who received their first lung cancer diagnosis between 1990 and 2013. These individuals with lung cancer had been hospitalized due to a serious mental illness as reported by the Hospital Discharge Register and recorded deaths were reported relative to this cohort from the Finnish Causes of Death statistics. To explicate the impact of serious mental illness on the rate of mortality, the team examined the competing risk analysis using the estimated hazard ratios (HRs).

Of the 37,852 lung cancer patients in Finland, 12% had a recorded history of serious mental illness and cancer-specific mortality rates were found to be differentiated between patients with certain types of cancer when factors such as stage of development of cancer at the time of representation and treatment were considered. The study showed that male cancer patients with squamous cell carcinoma who had a history of psychosis constituted the highest category of mortality risk whereas a comparable risk was noted among female cancer patients suffering from psychosis having small-cell carcinoma. A similarly high risk was found among female cancer patients suffering from psychosis and mood disorders in adenocarcinoma. The findings were clearly indicative of patients suffering from serious mental illness with elevated cancer-specific mortality. These findings called for a rededication to a collaborative endeavor combining patients, mental healthcare workers and oncologists if issues related to efforts at reducing the mortality disparity in rates between patients with serious mental illness and those without SMI were to be effectively addressed.

An essential characteristic of science is the on-going need for research wherein the science is able to develop and mature within the spectrum of collaborative research and funding. Thanks to the emergence of the U.S. National Institutes of Health better than half a century ago, a massive amount of federal funding of research has been and is being realized. Though private funding of scientific research, specifically medical research, has a history reaching back into the middle of the 19th century, only since the middle and late 20th century has the funding been so significant in size and breadth as to have transformed the face of medical science throughout the world. Much of the leading cancer research funding goes to the outstanding centers who have distinguished themselves in break-through databased research. The Mongan

Institute of the Massachusetts General Hospital, a Harvard Medical School affiliate, is one of the most significant in this field of research. Efren J. Flores of the Mongan Institute has put together an outstanding panel of Institute colleagues for the purpose of exploring the feasibility and acceptability of lung cancer screening relative to patients suffering from serious mental illness (Flores, Neil, Tiersma, Pappano, et al., 2021). They were particularly focused on the issue of a collaborative educational intervention program designed specifically for this particular cancer population. Might it be possible, they asked, to design an educational intervention screening program for lung cancer patients suffering from a mental illness which could prove both doable (feasible) and worthy of the effort (acceptable).

Confident in their own professional capabilities in developing more refined research tools and in response to the documented reality that there exists universally a major disparities in survival rates among lung cancer patients suffering from a serious mental illness versus those patients who do not have this comorbidity. Therefore, this talented team of oncology researchers developed an educational intervention tool (called Phase 1) using a two-phase, mixed-methods approach in the creation of a person-centered lung cancer screening (LCS) tool specifically for cancer patients suffering from schizophrenia and a bipolar disorder (SMI). They then employed this screening tool in order to evaluate acceptability, feasibility, and measurable changes in patients' attitudes towards the LCS tool (called Phase 2).

In the development of Phase 1 of this massive study, the team used three focus groups joined by professionals in the fields of mental health, primary care, and radiology in their assessment of rapid qualitative analysis. Designed specifically for patients suffering from a serious mental illness (primarily schizophrenia and bipolar disorder but not excluding paranoia), the focus was upon LCS intervention (walk-through video and smoking cessation handouts). Phase 2, then, engaged in the actual enrollment of LCS-eligible cancer patients suffering from a serious mental illness (n=15) wherein the team assessed the feasibility and acceptability of this designed LCS educational intervention instrument conducted by a radiologist and a mental health professional at a community mental health clinic. Cancer patients participating in this study were observed relative to attitudes regarding lung cancer itself, the LCS instrument and usage, and, interestingly enough but most insightful, tobacco smoking before and following the LCS intervention.

The analysis of the findings of this study centered round a two-phase response. Phase 1, consisting of three categories of participants, viz., primary care physicians, radiologists, and mental health clinicians, in which there was a consensus of response that a person-centered language was desirable as well as the use of an instructive video showing how the process of the LCS actually addressed personal concerns of patients with a severe mental illness. Phase 2, then, showed that 50% of the participating patients actually enrolled in the LCS intervention scheme with 100% completing the intervention with only 7% of the participants registering dissatisfaction with the experience. However and a point of concern was the fact that the participants in this study reported a rise in their personal worry regarding the possibility of developing lung cancer following the intervention protocol. The team called for an accelerated collaboration between radiologists and primary care providers in a community mental health clinic in order to enhance the efforts in the LCS instrument use for patients suffering from SMI.

Throughout this study, we have identified an imprecise sliding scale of definitional terms used to describe mental illness and psychiatric disorders such that the range of applications of the SMI description covers everything from mild depression and anxiety to paranoid schizophrenia! In each databased study which we have explored in this work, the researchers are keen to actually identify and circumscribe the mental illness which they are studying such that there is usually little or no confusion within the research team as to what is actually being investigated. However, the definitional envelope is somewhat expanded beyond common usage in the case of studies focusing upon the relationship between trauma and cancer. Tyler S. Kaster of the faculty of medicine (psychiatry) at the University of Toronto (Canada) has been joined by several medical professionals from his own university as well as from the University of Manitoba to sort out the relevance of studies of Post-traumatic stress and cancer using a cross-sectional nationally representative sample (Kaster, Sommer, Mota, Sareen, El-Gabalawy, 2019). This study constitutes one of the earliest and most comprehensively detailed investigations into the relationship of PTSD and the various types of cancer linked to this disorder. Moving beyond the popular focus upon PTSD related to military experience, this team expanded its scope of consideration to include a range of traumatic factors and covering both male and female cancer patients. This team points out at the beginning of this research that though there have been a number of distinguished studies done on the relationship of patients suffering from PTSD who have various physical conditions, there has been very little attention given to the relationship of PTSD to patients with cancer. This study was designed to address that deficiency in research.

Focusing their attention upon 36,309 patients identified by a cross-sectional National Epidemiologic Survey on Alcohol and Related Conditions (NESARC) for 2012-2013, the team investigated the linkage between trauma, PTSD and cancers of breast and gastrointestinal as well as a wider range of unspecified cancer types. These 36,000+ respondents to the survey were classified as no-trauma, trauma-exposed, and PTSD based on definitional parameters established by the DSM-5 (*Diagnostic and Statistical Manual of Mental Disorders, 5TH edition).* They employed the non-trauma exposed category of respondents as a reference point for conducting both cancer and sex stratified regression analyses attempting to circumscribe the linkage between PTSD and cancer patients. What the team discovered was that there was a much greater presence of cancer in PTSD respondents than in those who were either trauma-exposed or no-trauma exposed without the diagnosis of PTSD but a greater trauma-exposed cancer rate than among no-trauma respondents. However, when there was an adjustment made for a range of covariates, the team discovered that there was a measurable increase of cancer in PTSD patients as over against the non-trauma-exposed respondents measuring for "any" type of cancer but with breast cancer proving of no significance. What proved most helpful in this analysis was the discovery with statistical verification that both males and females with PTSD were much more susceptible to all kinds of cancers than non-PTSD respondents. Even the differentiation across sexes demonstrated that those who had been trauma exposed were more likely to develop cancer than non-trauma exposed. In the final analysis the team's conclusion was that an exposure to trauma and PTSD were clearly linked to cancer though they were able to determine that the comorbid linkage between traumatic exposure, PTSD, and cancer varied measurably based on sex and cancer type. The study clearly called for more research on the relationship of trauma to cancer.

Geriatric oncological psychiatry constitutes a fundamental manifestation of a tripartite assessment and treatment agenda wherein the elderly patient suffering from cancer is brought into the matrix of a psychiatric evaluation. Efi Parpa and colleagues at School of Medicine of the University of Athens in Greece provided an admirable assessment and evaluation of 102 medical journal publications coupled with a comprehensive search of databases covered in PubMed and PsychINFO (1980-2013) wherein the key search words proved most productive, i.e., such terms as "cancer", "elderly", "aging", "geriatric", "psychiatric disorders", "psychiatric symptoms", "psychological problems", "aged >60 years", "suicidal ideation, geriatric, cancer", "suicide geriatric cancer" (Parpa, Tsilika, et al., 2015). The review of published research scholarship constitutes one of the most important methods of accessing current work in a medical field as illustrated in Morgan's (2023) work titled *Cancer and Suicide: A Resource Compendium of Published Research (1978-2023).* Parpa and team were clear about the intention of this research project for they were focused on establishing to what extent there is a relationship between elderly cancer patients and psychiatric health such that both the oncology community as well as the psychiatric community might be more thoroughly informed.

Within the classification types of mental illness universally recognized is that of depression and this team illustrated just how commonly manifested this mental health issue is present in the geriatric community wherein cognate features most frequently present are disability, morbidity, and mortality. Often linked to depression is that of the experience of anxiety which is somewhat less evident in the early stages of geriatric cancer but with the increasing of age anxiety becomes ever more apparent. Parpa's team clearly validated the realization that psychiatric disorders are commonly evidenced in geriatric patients suffering from cancer and the overall intention of this study was to call attention to this reality and to appeal to the health care community to be ever more attentive to the coupling of geriatric cancer and mental illness with an eye towards the enhancement of quality care of the patient as well as that of the personal attention to the care givers themselves.

Psychiatry has an extended history of concern for the mental health patient who has overcome a psychiatric disorder and the tracking of the post-treatment overall behavior and well-being of the post-psychiatric patient constitutes an ongoing area of research and study. Oncologists likewise have an enduring interest in the overall behavior and well-being of the post-cancer patient for there is the general recognition that among both post-psychiatric and post-cancer patients there is always the possibility of a return of the disorder. The study of post-treatment survivorship has emerged as a major field of databased study in recent years whether the patient is a survivor of surgery, cancer, or a mental disorder. Surviving a traumatic encounter with a potentially terminal illness often results in the emergence of other debilitating issues affecting behavior and general well-being. The sophistication of survivorship research is reflected in the specificity of topic such that a study of lung cancer and survivorship may have some points of commonality with breast cancer but the more refined the database search is the more important and insightful the findings may prove to be.

Such is the case with a study of mental illness among ovarian cancer patients who reach the point of survivorship. Clearly, an ovarian cancer survivor confronted with mental illness constitutes a legitimate focus of research for oncologists and psychiatrists alike and certainly comes within the domain of psychiatric oncology.

Because ovarian cancer is the 5th most common cancer among women, there is a need to pay closer attention to the issues related to survivorship and the relevance of a mental illness during and after cancer treatment. The ever-present prospects of suicidality as well as debilitating depression are causes for medical concern. Siqi Hu of the Huntsman Cancer Institute in Salt Lake City (UT) has put together a team of medical researchers from the Huntsman Cancer Institute as well as the University of Utah School of Medicine precisely to address the research challenge of better understanding issues related to ovarian cancer survivorship with mental illness (Hu, Baraghoshi, Chang, Rowe, et al., 2023). Databased studies of ovarian cancer patient survivorship with accompanying mental illness are rare and inconclusive beyond generalized surmises regarding on-going health care issues. Hu and colleagues set about the solidify findings on this topic based on a substantial databased research project. This project was two pronged in that it first determined to explore the incidence of mental illness among ovarian cancer survivors relative to the general population but also secondly to examine the risk factors for mental illness among ovarian cancer survivors. This two-pronged research project proved to be ground breaking in survivorship studies.

The initial data was comprised of a cohort of 1,689 ovarian cancer patients who had been diagnosed with cancer between the years 1996 and 2012 with 7,038 women matched by age and birth who did not have cancer. The diagnosis of mental illness was based on electronic medical records as well as statewide healthcare facilities which provided relevant data. Cox proportional hazard models were used in the estimated hazard ratios relative to the cohort data base. What the team learned from this large data base was that women who survived ovarian cancer actually experienced an elevated risk of mental illness within the first 2 years following the cancer diagnosis. The risk of a debilitating depression within the cohort of women survivors of ovarian cancer was almost 3-fold higher the first 2 years of the initial cancer diagnosis and just shy of 2-fold between 2 and 5 years following the diagnosis. What proved most enlightening and disturbing was the discovery that women surviving ovarian cancer encounter an 80% elevated risk of death if they were suffering from a mental illness and over 90% increased risk of death if they had been diagnosed with a debilitating depression.

It fell the responsibility of this research team to conclude that elevated and increased risks of mental illness could be noted within the cohort of ovarian cancer survivors throughout the entire follow-up periods of up to 5 years following the cancer diagnosis. Therefore, there was a call for a multidisciplinary care protocol in both the monitoring and treating of mental illness within the ranks of ovarian cancer survivors.

In our discussion of databased studies of cancer over the past five years we have been consistently reminded of the disparities of quality of care and treatment involved in oncological practice often directly affected by such key factors as the mental state of the patient, age, geography, economic standing, etc. There has yet emerged as validated model of consistency in service to a broad spectrum of cancer patients.

One area of extreme disparity is evidenced in the databased studies related to the mental health of the cancer patient. All other variables aside, the care of serious mental illness (SMI) among cancer patients shows an issue of a higher mortality rate than within the general population. Kelly E. Irwin of the Department of Psychiatry at the Massachusetts General Hospital in Boston has launched a databased investigation into this issue of disparity between serious mental illness and cancer. Joined by a large number of outstanding oncologists and psychiatric professionals from Massachusetts General Hospital and Harvard Medical School, this research project focused upon the possibility of a person-centered collaborative care treatment plan designed specifically for cancer patients with serious mental illness. It was thought that this effort might prove helpful in addressing this international disparity (Irwin, Park, Fields, Corveleyn, et al., 2019).

This research team believed that psychiatric care of the cancer patient offered directly in conjunction with the diagnosis at the time of assessment might actually improve the overall outcome of treatment. At the time of this study there were no recognized models of verification demonstrating the a consistent effectiveness in conjoining psychiatry and cancer care. Therefore, this research team set out to explore the viability of what they chose to call a person-centered collaborative care trial for cancer patients suffering from serious mental illness, a methodology they labelled the "Bridge" designed to integrate psychiatric assessment and cancer treatment modalities. They focused their psychiatric interest in schizophrenia, bipolar disorder, and severe major depression. *(Note: As has been discussed at length earlier in this review of literature, the distinction between "serious" mental illness and "severe" mental illness has proven irrelevant though it should be pointed out that PubMed lists the latter twice as frequently as the former but this MGH research team chose to use the former throughout their study and so will we in this review of their work.)*

The design of Bridge as explained by the research team was built upon a tripartite constellation of factors consisting of (1) identification of patients with serious mental illness (SMI), (2) psychiatric and case management based on person-centered care, and (3) collaborative engagement with oncological practice. The team's initial study covered 12 weeks of a single group of patients suffering from SMI having just been diagnosed with breast, gastrointestinal, lung, or head/neck cancer. There was a three-step method of assessment of Bridge as an effective tool. First, the researchers considered the factors of cancer patient identification, enrollment and completion of the process. They then assessed the proposed benefits of this process by means of exit interviews involving patients, caregivers, and oncologists. Finally, they evaluated measurable change in psychiatric symptomatology using the Brief Psychiatric Rating Scale (BPRS).

Over a six month period from fall of 2015 to spring of 2016, there were 24 patients assessed of which 23 reported their meetings with the psychiatrist meaningful while 19 caregivers indicated that Bridge did speak to significant challenges faced by the caregivers. Oncologists involved in this study of the effectiveness of Bridge reported that for nearly 95% of their patients it proved either "very" or "most" useful. In addition to reporting that psychiatric symptoms on the BPRS actually improved, the team also noted that the exit interview involving all groupings of participants – patients, caregivers, oncologists – led to the observation that Bridge did foster patient-clinician trust while increasing accessibility to psychiatric care and treatment which then facilitated the patients' ability to complete their cancer treatments. This team of researchers called for randomized trials for the purpose of evaluating the overall value of this approach to the cancer care of an acutely underserved population of cancer patients suffering from serious mental illness. They were convinced, based on this study, that Bridge constitutes a viable and effective care delivery model for this category of cancer patients as well as of real benefit to the caregivers and oncologist, involved in the overall care of this category of patients.

In long-term treatment of cancer from diagnosis to mortality, one of the greatest challenges for the oncology team is determining to what extent the patient is able to actually participate in decisions related to treatment and protocol when the patient is not only suffering from cancer but is susceptible to mental illness and psychiatric disorder. It is universally documented within the oncology community that patients suffering from a serious mental illness are subject to a poorer survival rate compared to cancer patients not suffering from an SMI when all other relevant variables are controlled for. The disparity in the patient's decision-making capacity places a great deal of responsibility on the treatment team when the cancer patient has a shared comorbidity between cancer and mental illness. Daniel C. McFarland of the Northwell Health Cancer Institute of Lenox Hill Hospital in New York put together a team of oncology professionals from his Institute and that the Memorial Sloan Kettering Cancer Center for the purpose of researching this heretofore commonly overlooked variable of mental illness and decision-making when it comes to equitable and beneficent care (McFarland, Voigt, Alicia, 2021). The impairment of the patient's decision-making capacity and the equitable character of the decisions made when dealing with a cancer patient suffering from a mental illness constitutes the fundamental focus and challenge of this research project. The research team was aware from the outset that both the decision-making capacity (DMC) and the shared decision making (SDM) constituted a combined factor of difficulty in making equitable treatment protocols and this comprised their research agenda.

In an effort to focus their research on a specific demonstration of the nature and function of the decision-making capacity of a cancer patient with mental illness, the research team concentrated their study of 97 hospitalized cancer patients in a single cancer care institution. The participating institution provided the researcher with information from their patients' medical records including their serious mental illness data, demographics and cancer-related variables of care and treatment. They then compared and contrasted descriptive data from patients both with and without decision-making capacity records using a logistic regression model. The results of this study of the psychiatric consultations for DMC in these 97 hospitalized cancer patients showed an overall 42% manifestation of a DMC not dissimilar from that of patients with SMI. This latter group of patients with a serious mental illness proved to be younger in age all the while receiving anticancer treatment and actually demonstrated less susceptible to end of life issues. Age and the absence of any recent anticancer treatments were significant in their linkage to decisional incapacity such that three months following release from the cancer hospital, nearly two-thirds had died without any measurable distinction from those surviving based on their serious mental illness. However, patients not suffering from a serious mental illness demonstrated a concern for end of life issues (EOL) upwards of 63% while those with a serious mental illness did so at only a 36% rate of reported concerns. What proved most interesting and helpful to the research team was the discovery that there was no measurable difference based on SMI for cancer patients suffering from healthcare proxy, four determinate of DMC, including repeated psychiatric assessments based on decision-making capacity.

This study demonstrated the ineffectiveness of using the shared decision making (SDM) instrument on cancer patients who are suffering with a serious mental illness which led the researchers to suggest that accelerated directives including an aggressive effort to demonstrate value-congruent care for cancer patients suffering from a serious mental illness with the aim of reducing the inequities found among SMI patients relative to the DMC.

Not only oncologists but epidemiologists are always cognizant of the need for quality access to treatment on a timely basis for patients diagnosed with cancer. This has always been an abiding concern among cancer treatment professionals especially as linked to rural counties. The correlation between quick and effective diagnosis and treatment and mortality has been established without question. The delay in diagnosis and treatment has a profound impact upon the mortality of the newly diagnosed cancer patient and when that diagnosed patient is also concurrently suffering from mental illness, the urgency of immediate and effective treatment is significantly accelerated. The need for the oncology community to be aware of the health care shortage areas with reference to accessibility to quality care is self-evident. Cole B. Haskins of the Department of Epidemiology at the College of Public Health in the University of Iowa has put together a team of health care professionals for the specific purpose of investigating the impact that diagnostic and treatment shortages have in rural counties in the U.S. labeled Health Professional Shortage Areas (HPSA) with particular attention to breast cancer hormonal (endocrine) therapy and its relationship to the possible effects of such diminished access has upon patients suffering concurrently with a mental illness (Haskins, McDowell, Carnahan, et al., 2021).

The challenge to any cancer patient under long-term treatment is adherence to the set protocol designed by the oncology team servicing the patient. Without a conscientious compliance to the directives of the treatment professional oncology team, the efficacy of the treatment is inevitably in jeopardy. Haskins and colleagues took a close databased look at recipients of breast cancer endocrine therapy with special attention to the impact variances in patient adherence had upon the at-risk cancer patient suffering also from mental illness. Covering a span from 2007 to 2013, the research team took a roster of patients identified by the SEER-Medicare database of 21,892 women over the age of 68 suffering from Stage I breast cancer. Taking the assessment of HPSA regarding the shortage of access to cancer care status, these patients' counties were categorized as least, moderate, and highest shortage of health care with counties for which there was no documentation and, therefore, were classified in a fourth category. The team used the Cox regression test for endocrine therapy initiation and discontinuation including an assessment of daily adherence with longitudinal linear regression for the 21,000+ patients being evaluated.

It was determined by the research team that based on the necessary multivariate adjustments, cancer patients who resided in primary care shortage counties were less likely to take the initiative in seeking endocrine therapy than otherwise. Counties falling outside the evaluated status as determined by the researchers more commonly had a higher rate of oncologists *per capita* and showed fewer residence who fell below the federal poverty level and higher incomes *per capita* than otherwise. However, they found that mental health shortages were actually not linked to cancer treatment outcomes. Patients living in these unevaluated counties were inclined to discontinue bipolar and psychotic disorders as well as substance abuse and anxiety disorders. Therefore, concluded the research team, there was a disinclination on the part of those living in such counties to initiate endocrine therapy treatment based on poor primary care access. They did discover that patients living in counties which were deficient in mental health care actually demonstrated a reduction in the harmful association between mental illness and incomplete cancer treatment. Patients who were diagnosed with mental illness, the team reasoned, may actually be better prepared to follow through with cancer treatment if they are given access to better mental health care such that a linkage of better primary care and mental health care seems evident.

Science is never finished with a research topic but always pursuing further the breadth and depth of the findings with an eye towards refinement, correction, and discovery. This is most decidedly the fundamental descriptive characteristic of medical research and it is particularly evident in cancer research as oncologists and cognate professionals continue to address nuanced applications of treatment protocols with the aim for perpetual improvement. In recognition of the documented reality that patients suffering from serious mental illness (SMI) who also have been diagnosed with cancer are particularly vulnerable to a disparity and inequity of care reflected in the elevated rate of cancer-specific mortality. Kelly E. Irwin of the Department of Psychiatry at the Massachusetts

General Hospital and Harvard Medical School was joined by a dozen health care professionals involved in oncological research related to the care and treatment of cancer patients suffering from serious mental illness (aka severe mental illness) with particular attention to a modality of care and treatment referred to as Bridge or person-centered collaborative care protocol (Irwin, Callaway, Corveleyn, Pappano, 2022).

This team began with the domain assumption that an integration of intentional mental health care early on at the time of a cancer diagnosis has the potential of improving the delivery of quality cancer care for those patients who are particularly suffering from a serious mental illness. However, access to this quality care is often problematic in terms of both availability and personnel equipped to deal with this matrix of health issues, i.e., both cancer and mental illness in a single patient. Concerned for the care of this particularly marginalized constituency of cancer patients suffering from mental illness, this research team set about to test the efficacy of a collaborative care approach to this category of patient which had not at the time of their study been systematically delineated and explicated relative to a specific specialized model of care called "Bridge."

This research team began their search for answers by a 24-week single-site randomized trial based on the person-centered collaborative care program (Bridge) designed for patients suffering from a range of severe mental illnesses such as schizophrenia, bipolar disorder, and major depression requiring psychiatric hospitalization including a study of their caregivers in this survey. The total participants were 120 patients randomized for Bridge or the EUC (Enhanced Usual Care) including the patients' caregivers. This research team engaged in a proactive identification of patients suffering from a serious mental illness including a new breast, lung, gastrointestinal, or head and neck cancer susceptible to curative treatment. The Enhanced Usual Care protocol included the specification that the oncologists of each patient be informed regarding the patient's psychiatric diagnosis as well as actually notifying patients about variously provided psychosocial services leading to a tracking of both the patient and caregiver outcomes.

On the other hand, Bridge involved a robust proactive assessment by psychiatrists and social workers constituting a person-centered team approach to overall assessments of patients including an orchestrated collaboration involving both mental health professionals and oncologists providing an elevated access to evidence-based psycho-oncology care. For purposes of this evaluative study of Bridge and EUC, the outcome sought was cancer care disruptions assessed by a blind panel of oncologists leading to an outcome assessment involving patient and caregiver-reported outcomes and healthcare accessibility and utilization. Using a mixed method of assessment, barriers to Bridge implementation and dissemination were scrutinized and evaluated. The overall characteristic of this projected evaluative trial of Bridge and EUC was designed to provide information reflective of efforts to carefully identify individuals suffering from serious mental illness and as well as cancer. The aim was to actually produced experimental evidence form evaluating the impact of person-centered collaborative care for this particularly underserved population.

The care of cancer patients with mental illness constitutes a monumental challenge to any health care facility and to the medical staff assigned to their care. Many studies have focused upon the perception of the cancer care situation from the point of view of the patient and often the patient's family as well and concerns over how the cancer diagnosis has exacerbated a potential mental crisis. Psychiatric oncologists are particularly attuned to the multiplicity of issues faced by a newly diagnosed cancer patient and are themselves especially aware of the eminent dangers of the patient developing a psychiatric disorder linked to or resulting from a cancer diagnosis. What is less commonly studied is that of the impact that a cancer diagnosis of a patient with a mental disorder has to that of the attending medical staff, psychiatrist, oncologist, nursing personnel and health care administrators. More needs to be known about the impact of this encounter faced by the medical team and not just issues relevant to the patient.

All oncologists and cancer care medical professionals are fully aware of the pervasive disparities and inequities which exist in the care of cancer patients and more particularly with those cancer patients suffering from a mental disorder. This reality is known and recognized throughout the world among all cognate professionals working with cancer patients. Though this knowledge is well known such information is more commonly recognized by the patient than by the personal provider and institutional care personnel. In a serious effort to address these disparities and inequities as perceived by the medical team itself, Yuto Yamada of the Department of Neuropsychiatry at the Okayama University Graduate School of Medicine in Japan has put together a distinguished team of likeminded medical professionals from a variety of Japanese medical institutions (Yamada, Fujiwara, Etoh, Wada, et al., 2022). Rather than focusing upon the care of the patient from the patient's point of view, Yamada and team have directed their examination to delineating the complex issues related to the medical professionals' own personal perceptions of the disparities and inequities in cancer patient care. The interest is specifically upon the difficulties of the care of cancer patients suffering from a mental illness as experienced by the medical team attending such patients.

Relying on contact information provided by 17 cancer hospitals in Japan, this research team designed and distributed a mail questionnaire focusing on 29 specific items related to the difficulties in the care of cancer patients with a mental disorder as well as an inquiry regarding the experienced insufficiencies in the medical protocol of treatment using a five-point Likert scale. The analytical classification of responses centered around the number of respondents who indicate "difficult/insufficient" in each of the 29 items under scrutiny with notes designating those respondents who indicated access to psychiatric support services within their hospitals. The response to the mailed questionnaire resulted in 388 (58.4%) cancer care providers responding to four delineated areas of concern reflected in the research instrument. These were (1) issues relevant to difficulties in the diagnosis and treatment of the patient's cancer, (2) the presence of support for the treatment decision-making factors, and (3) the overall assessment of the patient's adherence to treatment protocols, with special attention to the assessment of the patient's physical symptoms perceived as most difficult for the medical personnel with which to address and manage (which represented upwards of 80% of the medical respondents' comments).

An most finding was that the most difficult collaborative factor among the multidisciplinary health care providers was the issue of advanced consultations as well as the sharing of patient information with the patient's primary psychiatric care team (representing 52.2% of respondents). Furthermore, issues involving the insufficiencies of in-hospital and community-based medical services were measured as most insufficient (47.4%) when it came to educating the patient regarding reasonable accommodations. It was the varying levels of psychiatric support which constituted the basis on which over half of the perceived difficulties from hospital to hospital were evidenced. In the final analysis, this research team suggested that some of these glaring difficulties regarding cancer care for patients with mental disorders as seen and understood by the cancer care providers might well be alleviated through a more robust psychiatric liaison among the medical service providers.

Both from the perspective of the psychiatric community and that of the oncology community, there is always the concern to determine to what extent, if any, there is an identification of factors linking mental illness to cancer. By dispelling any notion that such a biochemical causal linkage exists constitutes a major advancement in the clinical research related to some form of identifying markers linking the statistics of cancer patients with mental illness. In the absence of any clinical evidence of a biochemical link between cancer and mental illness, verified over and over again in clinical laboratory tests and statistical analysis of international data bases, the research community is at liberty to move towards the driving agenda of psychiatric oncology which focuses upon the psychosocial spectrum of cancer care (Morgan, 2023). Elizabeth Siantz of the Family Medicine and Public Health Department of the University of California in San Diego was joined in her research initiative by faculty members from the Keck School of Medicine at the University of Southern California to further explore the clinical and statistical reports that mental illness does not manifest any linkage with patient adherence to colorectal cancer screening based on data provided by the California Health Interview Survey (Siantz, Wu, Shiroiski, Vora, and Idos, 2017).

Factors identified by the research team which precipitated this monumental databased study including the fact that in the U.S. colorectal cancer constitutes the second leading cause of cancer-specific death combined with the fact that individuals suffering from mental illness (including unspecified types), actually receive less preventive health care services such as specifically cancer screening. The domain assumption on the part of the researchers was formed as a hypothesis that suggested that mental illness constitutes a fundamental risk factor for patients not complying with colorectal cancer-screening guidelines. This they set out to test in a major databased study involving the analysis of records provided by the 2007 California Health Interview Survey of individual patients aged 50 years old and older (N=15,535). This test was designed to determine whether and to what extent, if any, mental illness presents a risk factor for patients not complying with colorectal cancer-screening recommendations. The team used weighted multivariate logistic regressions and identified mental illness based on the Kessler K 6 screening tool. Data was representative of the State of California's population and screening was circumscribed as either fecal occult blood testing for the previous year before testing and sigmoidoscopy or colonoscopy during the previous 5 year period. This study showed that mental illness could not be factually linked with colorectal cancer-screening compliance on the part of the patient and that risk factors for such non-adherence was particularly characteristic of female patients who delayed accessing health care for the previous year of the study.

A major concern registered by the researchers was the fact that earlier such studies occasionally suggested a link between mental illness and cancer-screening compliance on the part of the patient but in this study there was no such evidence. They accounted for the possibility of differences between their study and previous ones by suggesting that may the research population was a variant as well as possibly state-specific healthcare policies might affect the execution of the research method and finding conclusions. Further studies of the California population were, therefore, called for by this research team.

A fundamentally important research method in medical science is that of comparisons between certain groups, particularly those with a disorder or illness and those without. In this way, it becomes clearer for researchers to actually identify those factors which might have contributed to the development of a disease in one group and not in another. In oncological research, the range of types of cancers is staggering and therefore to focus research attention upon one type of cancer as compared to individuals without cancer constitutes a standard operational procedure. Beyond just determining contributory factors in the differentiation between those with a certain type of cancer and those without, a further refinement of this targeting research method is to enquire into the nature and function of the actual cancer screening of both groups. In the case of a major research undertaken led by B.J.H. Yarborough of the Kaiser Permanente Northwest Center for Health Research in Portland, Oregon (USA), there was a further interest in comparing two different screening methods related to colorectal cancer screening for both individuals with and without mental illness but who had colorectal cancer. Yarborough was joined by colleagues from the Portland research institution and from Johns Hopkins University in Baltimore, Maryland (USA), to address the rates of colorectal cancer (CRC) screening of cancer patients with and without a psychiatric disorder (Yarborough, Hanson, Perrin, Stumbo, Green, 2018) and to discover to what extent one screening program is either more effective than another or contributes to a combined effectiveness beyond single use methods.

What has made this study so significant in the field is the team's efforts at comparing two types of CRC screening tests, i.e., guaiac fecal occult blood testing (gFOBT) and fecal immunochemical testing (FIT) upon completing the CRC screening by some 92,445 general population cohorts based on a secondary analysis of generally available data. They conducted this study in a health system servicing nearly half a million members in urban and suburban communities in Oregon and Washington State. All participants involved in this study were themselves health system members and were sorted on the basis of mental illness diagnoses such as psychotic disorders, non-psychotic unipolar depression, and those with no mental illness documented at all. The participants were age-eligible and at average risk of CRC at least one year and a day beyond their past gFOBT showing no evidence of any other CRC screening experience.

The research team used Cox proportional hazard models and in their study found that the FIT test actually reduced CRC screening impediments for all participants. Participant members of the cohort who registered a psychotic disorder were as likely to participate in screening using FIT as those diagnosed with depression based on a comparison with individuals without any diagnosed mental illness. The research team was able to demonstrate that fecal immunochemical testing may effectively increase the CRC screening rates of patients with mental illnesses and psychiatric disorders and especially among patients with diagnosed depression.

A continuing field of specialization in oncology research has to do with the relationship of severe mental illness to differing types of cancer and not least of these relationships is that of mortality among individual patients suffering from colorectal cancer who also have been diagnosed with severe mental illness (SMI). In this specialized research field, some countries have put forth great effort in attempting to understand the complexities of this relationship and among those countries leading the way is that of Finland's National Institute for Health and Welfare in Helsinki. Kristiina Manderacka of that Institute has been joined by several of her colleagues at the Institute in Helsinki as well as researchers from the faculty of social sciences at the University of Tampere in Finland with the intention of focusing upon the history of SMI on mortality among patients suffering from colorectal cancer. Manderbacka has been joined in this registry-based cohort study by other oncologists and social scientists in a databased study producing insightful results (Manderbacka, Arffman, Lumme, Suvisaari, et al., 2018). Though acknowledging the fact that the linkage between psychiatric disorders and cancer generally has been exhaustively researched and data on the subject is extensive, this team was eager to emphasize the importance of a focus upon the direct relationship between severe mental illness (SMI) and specifically colorectal cancer (CRC) with particular interest in the history of SMI among such patients.

While using Cox regression models for recording the impact on SMI relative to mortality, the research team drew data from the Finnish Cancer Registry for the purpose of identifying patients whose first colorectal cancer diagnosis fell between 1990 and 2013 (n=41,708). They further researched hospital admissions based on a diagnosis of a severe mental illness which actually occurred prior to the cancer diagnosis (n=2,382). Finally, records from the Hospital Discharge Register and deaths from the Causes of Death statistics rounded out the statistical scope of this Finnish national study. The team found that with patients having a history of psychosis and (parenthetically, a substance use disorder as well), there was an elevation of colorectal cancer mortality compared to the general population and when their research model controlled for age, comorbidity, and the stages at presentation and treatment of cancer, mortality among male patients who had a history of psychosis experienced an elevation of mortality risks above that of women in the same cohort. Male patients manifesting substance use disorders also proved an excessive mortality rate.

Manderacka's research team registered a cautionary observation that more databased research is needed when addressing the issues involved in factors associated with the elevation of mortality among patients with a diagnostic history of psychosis as well as that of substance use. They called for more detailed clinical research emphasizing collaborative engagement pf patients, health care workers, and oncologists interested particularly in this field of study.

Though lung cancer is the first type of cancer death in the U.S., colorectal cancer comes in third for men and second for women and the call for further study of the relationship between CRC and mental health disorders continues unabated. We have explored a number of such studies relating mental health disorders to the prevalence of lung cancer but to broaden the oncological community's understanding of this complex relationship between cancer and mental health, Shane Lloyd of the Radiation Oncology Department of the university of Utah School of Medicine's Huntsman Cancer Institute has been joined by a substantial team of colleagues to specifically investigate further using a comprehensive database to delineate the nature of the relationship between colorectal cancer and mental health disorders relative to survival rates (Lloyd, Baraghoshi, Tao, et al., 2019). Increasingly, the oncology medical community has become aware of the absolute relevance of the psychosocial spectrum of cancer care such that embracing concerns relative to mental health and mental illness constitute a profoundly important overall component of cancer assessment, diagnosis, and treatment.

A particularly insightful research consideration by Lloyd and colleagues was a concern for understanding the survival rate of colorectal cancer patients (CRC) covering a spectrum from short-term to long-term periods of assessment in order to identify the actual risk factors for the appearance of mental illness among diagnosed CRC survivors. Using the Utah Cancer Registry for identifying CRC survivors, they focused on individuals diagnosed with colorectal cancer between the years 1997 and 2013. Thanks to a database linkage with the Utah Population Database (UPD), the team was able to identify mental health diagnoses using the UPD's electronic medical records and statewide facilities database. Since the aim was to compare CRC survivors with individuals in the general population cohort who did not have this type of cancer, the team pointed out that the risk of developing a mental illness was compared between those with and those without CRC. The linkage between mental illness and the mortality rate was also analyzed.

Of the nearly 36,000 individuals in the general population (n=35,897), nearly 9,000 colorectal cancer survivors were finally identified (n=8,961) and in this particular analysis the team found that the CRC survivors were actually at an elevated risk for the diagnosis of mental illness within the first 2 years of cancer identification and diagnosis. These same

CRC survivors were recognized as at an elevated risk of developing depressive disorders during the same time frame. Even after 5 years of diagnosis this risk remained high. The research showed that those factors linking an elevated risk of mental health disorders among the CRC survivors included particularly colostomy and the Charlson Comorbidity Index with an increased risk of mortality for the CRC survivors who had been diagnosed with any type of mental disorder including depression. Therefore, this research demonstrated that CRC survivors continued at an elevated risk of developing mental disorders in both the short-term and long-term with a much higher rate of mortality than the general population.

The identification, assessment, diagnosis and treatment of cancer has a long and distinguished history. The American Cancer Society became actively involved in encouraging screening for breast cancer in the late 1970s and the technology developed (and still being developed) for screening has exponentially accelerated the effectiveness of cancer screening and early identification of cancer. However, there is still an enduring challenge for oncologists to secure screening compliance particularly among cancer patients who also suffer from a mental disorder, particularly severe mental illness (SMI) or a substance use disorder (SUD). Studies have consistently shown a decline in cancer mortality when linked with cancer screening. Since colorectal cancer (CRC) is the third leading cause of cancer deaths in the U.S. and since screening has been credited with a decline in CRC mortality, it seems appropriate to increase attention on this process relative to the under-served mentally ill and substance abuse patients.

Focusing on the problems of a lower utilization of cancer screening by patients suffering from mental illness and substance abuse, Carolina Abuelo of Massachusetts General

Hospital and Harvard Medical School has been joined by a distinguished panel of institutional colleagues to focus attention precisely upon this disparity in screening behavior with particularly attention given to a developed patient navigation program on CRC screening for this special group of cancer patients in an attempt to determine to what extent there is a measurable effect on the rate of survival within this category of cancer patients (Abuelo, Ashburner, Atlas, et al., 2020). This team used a randomized control trial from January to June of 2017 from an urban area's health care center serving a low-income community of 251 cancer patients ranging in age from 50 to 74 years who suffered from a mental illness or substance use diagnosis who were subject belatedly to a CRC screening. These patients were either subjects of intervention or a usual stratified care suffering from mental illness, an SUD, or both.

The process of implementation of this study was built around a focus on intervention group of patients who received a written communication followed by a phone call from the designated patient navigators. The function of the navigator was to facilitate patient compliance after addressing personal concerns and anxieties regarding the CRC screening. This included such resistant variables as patient education, problems with scheduling, instructions in bowel preparation, and problems with transportation for appointments. In those cases in which the patient was resistant to a colonoscopy it fell the responsibility of the patient navigator to offer the alternative use of a fecal occult blood testing. The challenge for the study was the level of full compliance by the patient in completing the requirements for the CRC screening.

Of the 251 originally identified cancer patients selected for this study, 85 (67%) of them were contacted directly by the appointed navigators in the intervention group with 26 actually refusing to become involved in this study. In an overall assessment of the analysis of treatment responses, the research team found that more of the patients involved in the intervention group actually received CRC screening (19%) than was true of the usual care group (10.4%). Of the 56 intervention patients subjected to navigation, 33+% actually completed the screening process as opposed to the control group (10.4%). The research team found, on the basis of this narrowly constructed study, that the patient navigation program (PNP) actually improved the CRC screening rates in both patients with mental illness and SUD. Clearly, a larger test employing these refinements to the study is needed to deepen the understanding of the effectiveness of this approach to this vulnerable patient grouping.

Thanks to the burgeoning sub-field of psychiatric oncology (aka psychosocial oncology) developed to specifically address the psychosocial spectrum of cancer care, there is a broad range of knowledge and interest in the dynamic relationship of the medical side of cancer care and the emotional side of cancer care. This dual approach should be treated as a unified composite of holistic medicine. From the early days of launching this field of applied cancer care under the leadership of Dr. Jimmie Holland at the Sloan-Kettering Cancer Institute and its medical journal, *Psychooncology,* a major focus of research has emerged in which the psychological and sociological side of the cancer patient's life has moved front and center in oncological studies and clinical practice. What has concerned clinicians in this development has been the overall impact that a diagnosis of cancer has upon the family unit itself, not just the patient but the support needed from the social matrix. Specialized research has grown in this area of interest such that psychiatric oncology is now recognized internationally as a *bona fide* specialization with its own rightful place in the composite of professional care central to the overall well-being of the patient and the patient's family.

Pushing the research deeper into the complexities of the relationship of a cancer diagnosis to the welfare of the patient and family unit, Jacqui van Warmerdam of the Children's hospital in Toronto, Canada, launched a databased study of the long-term mental health issues related to mothers and siblings of children diagnosed with cancer with special attention to the psychosocial impact over time such a development in the family matrix produces. Warmerdam was joined by several medical professionals from the Hospital for Sick Children and colleagues from the University of Toronto to conduct a monumentally significant databased study of this commonly overlooked feature of cancer care (Warmerdam, Sutradhar, Kurdyak, et al., 2020). This research team was fully cognizant of the central importance of the care of the mother and siblings of the diagnosed child cancer patient if the health of both the patient and the family were to fall within the spectrum of overall care.

The approach focused upon a childhood cancer registry in Ontario covering a span of time from 1998 to 2014 linking the birth records of a population-based cohort of mothers and siblings of children diagnosed with cancer. The mother and sibling cohorts (MSC) were arranged so as to correspond to a population control group linked to health care services data. The complexity of this comparative medical records study of patient, mother, and siblings required that the rate of mental health related outpatient visits (such as to a family physician and/or a psychiatrist) was companioned with the frequency of severe psychiatric episodes involving psychiatric emergency department visits, psychiatric hospitalizations, and even suicide) allowing for a comparison of mothers and siblings with the control group. Demographics, characteristics of the cancer patient, and oncology treatments were considered and examined as predictors of mental health outcomes.

This database was expansive for 4,773 mothers and 7,897 siblings of children who were diagnosed with cancer during the period 1998 to 2014 were compared to a control cohort in which both the mothers and siblings actually manifested an elevated rate of outpatient visits. However, the risk of severe psychiatric events did not increase in spite of the frequency of visits. The research team found that for mother and siblings, the demographic factors linked to a rise in the risk of adverse mental health issues included the younger material age at the time of the cancer diagnosis, a recognized low socioeconomic status of the family, and the rural residence characterizing the mother and older siblings of the patient. Though they found that certain mental health issues centered around the patient's family, treatment variables related to the cancer patient did not appear to be linked with other mental health outcomes of the patient. The team found that both mothers and siblings of the cancer patients actually experienced an elevation and an extended period of need for mental health care compared to the general population. Clearly, they found that demographic risk factors actually predicted the highest levels of risk within the patient's family matrix. The team was insistent that these data verified the legitimacy of a call for an intensification of psychosocial support and care of the child cancer patient's family members during the cancer treatment period and follow-up.

In the justifiable absence of any international body attempting to control the definition of medical terms, there is a general consensus within that massive community of professionals to agree to disagree about the nuanced parameters of certain medical terms so long as the intent and scope of the term is treated with integrity. Fortunately, the psychiatric community has not been encumbered by the ambiguities of nuanced usage of such terms as serious mental illness, severe mental illness, severe mental disorder, psychiatric disorder, and severe psychiatric illness. The research team chose to focus on the generally agreed upon application of all of these terms to a constellation of psychological manifestations of an emotional disturbance in the patient such that normally understood social functions are impaired or impeded. In recent decades, issues related to severe psychiatric illness has been deferred to the jurisdiction of psychiatric oncologists and to psychopathologists specializing in the psychosocial spectrum of cancer care when the treatment of a cancer patient exemplifying debilitating emotional dysfunction is present. Alyson L. Mahar of the Department of Community Health Sciences at the University of Manitoba has put together a team of likeminded colleagues from her own university as well as faculty from the ICES, the University of Toronto, and Queen's University to specifically investigate the effects on cancer treatment and mortality when the patient is being treated for colorectal cancer while suffering from a severe psychiatric illness (Mahar, Kurdyak, Hanna, Coburn, Groome, 2020).

As Mahar and colleagues have shown in this databased study of the relationship between cancer and mental illness, there is an enduring area of concern regarding the disparities and the apparent inequities in the survival rate of patients suffering from both as it raises questions regarding the nature and scope of the treatment protocol for the comorbidity of these patients. This research team's goal was twofold, namely, to identify the disparities and inequities of care reflected in the survival rates and them to examine closely the differences in treatment protocols as determined by the medical professionals. Is it possible that treatment plans of a cancer patient are conditioned by the cancer patient's mental health? This constituted the abiding question and concern of the Mahar research project and the resources at their disposal were quintessential in facilitating a deeper understanding of survival issues in the universal health care system in Ontario. Thanks to the resources of the ICES (Institute for Clinical Evaluative Sciences), this research team was able to launch a population-based retrospective cohort study linking data from the cancer registry as well as administrative data.

This databased research covered a period from April 1, 2007 to December 31, 2012 focusing on colorectal cancer patients suffering from severe psychiatric illness. The history of these patients' diagnosis constituted an address to those clinical descriptions included in the severe psychiatric illness (SPI) designation particularly including schizophrenia, schizoaffective disorders, unspecified psychotic disorders, bipolar disorders and other major depressive disorders. Patient history was based on hospitalization records, emergency department reports, and recorded psychiatric visits categorized as "no history of mental illness," "outpatient SPI history," and "inpatient SPI history." The intent of this research was to measure cancer-specific survival rates, non-receipt of surgical resections, and non-receipt of adjuvant chemotherapy or radiation. The statistical scope of this databased study was impressive covering 24,507 colorectal cancer patients of which 482 (2%) had an outpatient SPI history with 258 (1%) having an inpatient SPI history.

What these detailed statistical analyses were able to demonstrate for the research team was that cancer patients suffering from a history of a serious psychiatric illness actually experienced a lower survival rate than colorectal cancer patients who had no recorded history of mental illness owing to the fact that these patients received less guideline recommended treatment. They further found that the hazard rate for cancer-specific deaths was greater than one and a half times higher for those patients with an inpatient SPI and one and a quarter times higher for cancer patients with an outpatient SPI history. Also, cancer patients at the stage II and stage III level of development who also had an inpatient serious psychiatric illness history were actually better than two times less likely to undergo potentially curative surgical resection and two times less likely also to undergo adjuvant radiation or chemotherapy. Not surprisingly but nevertheless with a note of disappointment was the discovery based on these data that cancer patients who had a history of serious psychiatric illness encountered a measurable inequality in the care of their colorectal cancer including reported survival rates within the universal healthcare system developed and provided by the Canadian government in Ontario. This research team called for an accelerated increase in both advocacy and making cancer care resources more readily available to patients with SPI.

A distinctive feature of cancer research internationally is the common practice of focusing a topical concern in one country such that the findings of any serious databased study may actually be able to make a specific contribution to the health and well-being of a particular country with, of course, the possibility of internationally relevant extrapolations of the findings. To delineate the specific demographic characteristics of a particular cancer in a single country has often proven most beneficial to government agencies in the extension of health care services to their national population. Melinda M. Protani of the School of Public Health at the University of Queensland in Australia has done precisely that putting together a research team of cancer specialists from several national research centers in Australia for the specific purpose of focusing research on the relationship between colorectal cancer and mental illness (Protani, Jordan, Kendall, Siskind, et al., 2021). The relevance of mental illness to mortality of cancer patients generally is a major field of study and the Protani team chose to specialize their planned research in this matrix by focusing specifically upon patients with colorectal cancer suffering from severe mental illness and the effect of that linkage to mortality drawing their database from the Australian National Bowel Cancer Screening Programme (NBCSP). Rather than reporting findings, this published article was a careful delineation of the methodology to be employed in this projected study in hopes that their approach to identifying the relevant variables in the linkage of cancer and mental illness might prove of benefit to researchers in other countries interested in the same matrix.

The research impetus for the planned launching of this project grew out of the recognition that colorectal cancer's death rate is substantially elevated in cancer patients suffering from a severe mental illness compared to the general population of that country. This team has suggested that a fundamental blocking of elevated screening relative to cancer care could actually be linked to on-going disparities among CRC patients' mortality when those same patients are suffering from severe mental illness (SMI). Comparing colorectal cancer patients who have a diagnosed severe mental illness with CRC patients without an SMI within the general population based on data provided by Australia's National Bowel Cancer Screening Programme (NBCSP) will allow this research team to investigate treatment protocols following a cancer diagnosis such that an assessment of treatment options might contribute to the variance is CRC mortality among SMI and non-SMI patients.

Drawing from linked administrative data available for a retrospective cohort study of Australians aged 50 to 74 after 1 January 2006 both with SMI and those without, the team planned to focus on assessing the identifiable distinctions in the screening protocol of cancer care patients. Antipsychotic medication prescription data will characterize the medical profile of patients with a serious mental illness who are enrolled in Australia's universal healthcare system (Medicare). Information involving patient data outcomes from NBCSP participation, follow-up colonoscopy, CRC incident, and CRC-cause and all-cause mortality as well as confounders will be assessed from national-based and state-based administrative health datasets. The demographic focus of their planned research will involve the entire population of New South Wales aged 50 to 70 years who will have a new diagnosis of CRC on or after the first of January of 2006. There will be an attempt to ascertain the examination stage of the diagnosed cancer and subsequent treatment in both those with a severe mental illness and those without such. Incidence rates and rate ratios for each will rely on the Poisson regression analysis. Owing to the confidential nature of the anticipated database documentation, ethics approval will be secured from the University of Queensland Human Research Ethics Committee, the Australian Institute of Health and Welfare Ethics Committee, as well as the data custodians from every Australian State/Territory.

Cancer screening and early detection has its own checkered history of development and adoption within the medical community. As early as the 1920s, there was a movement to introduce screening for Pap test led by George

Papanicolaou who first applied this new procedure to cervical cancer and though initially the medical community was reluctant to embrace this new approach (not an uncommon characteristics of the traditionalism in medical practice) following the American Cancer Society's endorsement of the test during the 1960s screening has become commonplace though not universally available to all cancer patients relative to their socioeconomic status, nationality, and particularly their mental health. Since the introduction of screening for cervical cancer, for example, the mortality rate has dropped 50%. Where there has been a lag in research has been in the relationship between cancer screening to mental illness and mortality. Though all forms of cancer are relevant in any discussion of mortality and the place of mental illness in the diagnostic matrix, Marie D. Jorgensen of the Department of Clinical Epidemiology at the Aarhus University Hospital of Aarhus University in Denmark has focused her research specifically on the relevance of colorectal cancer screening to mental illness and has been joined by her University colleagues and faculty from the Department of surgery at the Randers Regional Hospital in Denmark (Jorgensen, Mikkelsen, Erichsen, Thomsen, 2022).

This research team began their research on the statistical reality that individuals with a mental illness have an elevated risk of colorectal cancer (CRC) mortality compared to the general population. They point out that it is possible that cancer screening for colorectal cancer may significantly reduce the mortality rate among this cancer group due to suffering from mental illness but documentation delineating to what extent this specific cancer group actually participates in CRC screening opportunities is limited. Jorgensen and colleagues chose to focus their research on a scoping review of the published medical literature which addressed the CRC screening of colorectal cancer patients suffering from mental illness. In order to comprehensively identify medical research published in the journals dealing with mental illness of patients participating in the CRC screening programs, this team examined the databases of PubMed, PsychInfo, Embase, and the Cochrane Library using only full-text papers published in English before February of 2021. For a refined focus of research on mental illness they chose to exclude published works in the journal literature dealing with dementia, intellectual disabilities, and developmental disabilities focusing rather specifically upon psychiatric disorders.

The researchers chose to classify the severity of mental illnesses reported in the 17 specific studies included in their scoping analysis. Cancer patients with a documented severe mental illness such as schizophrenia and bipolar disorder were actually less inclined to participate in the CRC screening made available to them as compared to the general population. Disappointing for the research was the indecisive findings regarding cancer patients suffering from common mental illnesses such as depression and anxiety and, therefore, the conclusions drawn from this literature analysis were assessed as insufficient for a clear understanding of the findings. This study was the first on record of a scoping review of the literature designed specifically to evaluate CRC screening program participation for cancer patients suffering from a diagnosed mental illness. Much future work is called for in light of the reality that the current medical literature is marginal in terms of the quality of findings since a large population based study is essentially required for a meaningful range of conclusions regarding the linkage between colorectal cancer patient screening and mental illness relative to mortality.

The professional staff of health care institutions and cancer treatment facilities is fully aware of the complex relationship between lifestyle and mental illness even though the nature of that relationship is uncertain and problematic. Complicating efforts to delineate the nature and scope of this relationship is the place of a cancer diagnosis in the mix. Psychiatric oncologists have for some time been aggressively highlighting the central importance of cancer care personnel and institutions concentrating more research focused on this tripartite matrix of cancer, mental illness, and lifestyle in order to more clearly understand the dynamics of those interactions with the aim of a reduction in the rate of mortality which characterizes this matrix. If a better understanding of the dynamics of this relationship can occur then oncologists, psychiatrists, and medical sociologists might more effectively collaborate in the development of a comprehensive treatment protocol addressing all three variables. Melinda M. Protani of the University of Queensland's School of Public Health in Australia has put together a team of medical faculty and health care professionals to precisely address issues related to the treatment of colorectal cancer patients suffering from a severe mental illness in order to better understand the high risk factors of mortality and to what extent lifestyle factors might play into a diagnosis regimen and treatment protocol (Protani, Alotiby, Seth, Lawrence, 2022). These research colleagues were chosen from a range of medical research facilities and institutions in Australia and were joined by faculty from the Department of Psychiatry at Dalhousie University in Canada.

From the outset the researchers were cognizant of the fact that patients suffering from a severe mental illness actually are susceptible to a higher risk of dying from colorectal cancer than the general population but were clear in their understanding that lifestyle factors seem not to be a determinant but they were unable to establish the differentiation between healthcare access and cancer treatment. Therefore, research designs employed by this team included cohort or population-based case-controlled designs and utilized full-text articles which were indexed in PubMed, EMBASE, PsychInfo, and CINAHL. These articles were specifically addressed to the comparisons of CRC treatment in patients both with and without pre-existing severe mental illnesses including specifically schizophrenia, schizoaffective, bipolar and major affective disorders. From the outset, the team sought to develop a systematic review and meta-analysis regarding access to guideline-appropriate care following a colorectal diagnosis in patients who suffered from severe mental illness including those who had undergone surgery, chemo- or radiotherapy.

The research team used ten carefully selected studies in which patients with severe mental illness experienced a reduced rate of a likelihood for surgery and though they realized that it was not possible to account for outcomes as shown by their meta-analyses. The actual results from variously selected individuals studies showed that patients with a severe mental illness were more commonly less inclined to receive radiotherapy, chemotherapy or sphincter-sparing procedures. The crucial discovery was that there existed a documented and measurably greater disparity in cancer care for patients suffering from a psychiatric disorder as inpatients than in the general population. The findings were conclusive in terms of disparity of care for patients suffering from severe mental illness (which included psychotic and affective disorders) were actually were the recipients of a deduced colorectal cancer care than that of the general public. The research teams believed this could be attributed to a higher case-fatality rate for patients with illnesses in places where the incidence of such is the same more or less as the general public. Reasons were merely speculative and led the research team to register a clarion call for more detailed study including a particular focus upon differences in treatment access and quality of care. This could possibly contribute to an excess colorectal mortality rate among patients suffering from a severe mental illness.

One of the great challenges for oncologists is securing consent from cancer patients to participate in a screening program and that challenge is further complicated if the cancer patient is suffering from a mental illness. Furthermore, recognizing that a mental disorder profoundly affects the willingness and readiness of a cancer patient is part of the challenge and when the cancer patient is suffering from colorectal cancer, there seems to be a greater level of resistance. Matte Kielsholm Thomsen in the Department of Clinical Epidemiology at the Aarhus University Hospital in Denmark has put together a team of oncologists and epidemiologists from within the University Hospital specifically to address the need for an evaluative assessment of the extent to which cancer patients suffering from mental disorders are willing to participate in a colorectal cancer screening program (Thomsen, Jorgensen, Pedersen, Erichsen, et al., 2023). The elevated rate of mortality among cancer patients suffering from a mental disorder is linked to colorectal cancer even though that rate is more or less comparable to that of the general population. The goal of this research team under the leadership of Jorgensen was to evaluate the evidence of cancer patients with a mental disorder's willingness to participate in a program of colorectal cancer screening in order that an assessment might be made of the effectiveness of the oncology community's utilization and promotion of such screening.

The team was able to identify from a national registry databank 2,036,704 Danish residents aged from 50 to 74 years old in a cohort study whom they invited to participate in a biennial fecal immunochemical testing between the dates of March 1, 2014 to September 30, 2018. Participation on the part of the test group was limited to a time period of 90 days from the time of the invitation to participate. They tracked the rate of participation of the cohort and assessed the screening results of the participants and their adherence to as well as the actual completion of a follow-up colonoscopy based on their mental disorder history (sorted according to none, mild, moderate, or severe). Of the initial databased cohort participants, 2,036,352 were finalized as the test cohort of whom 1,008,045 (49.5%) were men, 1,028,307 (50.5%) were women all with a mean age of just over 60 years (ranging from 49 to 78) but there was no data available for a determination of ethnicity. The researchers found that over against individuals with no reported or documented mental disorders, their analysis actually showed a diminished participation rate among individuals with either mild or moderate mental disorders. Participants with a severe mental disorder history were at 13.8% of the cohort members tested. These individuals with a recognized mental disorder actually demonstrated an elevated proportion of positive fecal immunochemical test results but with a somewhat lower adherence to colonoscopy than participants without a recorded mental disorder.

In the final analysis of their data, the team was able to show that individuals with a reported mental illness were actually less inclined to participate in a colorectal cancer screening as compared to individuals without a mental illness. However, they did emphasize that patients suffering from a mental disorder might significantly benefit from cancer screening if they were to receive a genuine and enthusiastic encouragement and support from their general practitioner or mental health care professional. A cautionary observation by the researchers suggested that the consideration of an intervention must take into account the type of mental disorder being experienced by the cancer subject to a colorectal screening as each situation is different.

In an earlier time in the mind of the general public, there was the false notion that if one had cancer (type unspecified) that was the beginning of the end. Even the designation of the type of cancer seemed not to have been a point of clarity. If it was cancer, that was all that needed to be said. In recent decades, the refinements in cancer types have been monumentally significant in determining the patient's life chances and certainly to focus the treatment of the diagnosis relative to the type of cancer involved. Combine the need to specify time within the framework of the mental health of the patient has become a fundamentally relevant ingredient in the assessment, diagnosis, and treatment of all types of cancer as well. Monique James of the Department of Psychiatry at the University of California's San Francisco (UCSF) Weill Institute for Neurosciences has put together a distinguished team of researchers from a range of leading institutions such as the Weill Institute, the Department of Medicine at the UCSF, and the College of Medicine at Florida Atlantic University specifically to address the relationship of cancer screening of women with cervical cancer suffering from severe mental illness (James, Thomas, Frolov, Riano, et al., 2017).

The focus was upon the screening rates for cervical cancer of women suffering from diagnosed severe mental illness and the data was provided by the California Medicaid Administrative (CMA) records for 2010-2011 which included a total of 31,308 women falling into this classification for whom medical records were available and accessible. Using the Poisson models for assessing the linkage between identified predictors and cervical cancer screening, participants in this study received special mental health services provided by the State of California and were not qualified under State guidelines for Medicare benefits. The results of this databased analysis was somewhat unanticipated for 20% of the women participants were suffering from severe mental illness who received cervical cancer screening during the one-year period of the study. Compared to White women in the study, Asian women, Black women, and Hispanic women were all more likely to have been screened than White women and women ages 28 to 37 were more likely to have been screened than women aged 18 to 27.

The most significant indicator of women's willingness to access cancer screening was whether or not they were taking advantage of other health care services. This fact constituted the strongest predictor of an inclination to seek screening. Because most women in this large databased study had not taken advantage of cervical cancer screening, there was a call for the research team for a more vigorous effort to aggressively promote such screening among this vulnerable population.

While the World Health Organization has as one of its primary goals the elimination of cervical cancer, there is a void in the knowledge of to what extent, if any, women suffering from mental illness actually comprise an identifiable group of patients at high-risk requiring prevention initiatives. This fact was effectively unknown prior to a study launched by Kejia Hu of the Department of Laboratory Medicine at the Karolinska Institutet in Stockholm, Sweden. Hu put together a distinguished international team of medical researchers to specifically address the absence of database studies investigating what his team chose to identify as invasive cervical cancer as well as precancerous lesions, and cervical screening engagement of Swedish women suffering from a mental illness (Hu, Wang, Sparen, Herweijer, et al., 2023). This Swedish research team was focused on the possible role of a prevention initiative aimed at women with cervical cancer concurrently suffering from a mental illness.

This group of researchers set out to determine whether women suffering from a severe mental illness, whether psychiatric or neurodevelopmental disorders, are more susceptible to an elevated risk of invasive cervical cancer as well as a rise in the risk of precancerous lesions accompanied by a decreased level of participation in cervical cancer screening as compared to women with a mental illness. This comparative study of risk among cancer patients was based on an observational study of 4,112,598 women patients from 1973 to 2018 in Sweden. The research focus addressed the issue of the risk of invasive cervical cancer, high-grade precancerous cervical lesions (CIN2), as well as the degree of participation in the cervical screening among women both with and without a mental illness. The study had a two-directional interest focusing upon both Severe Mental Illness (i.e., diagnosed in specialized psychiatric care) as well as a Milder Mental Illness (MMI) such as is used in psychotropic medications during primary care without specialist diagnosis. Using a nested case-control studies approach, the team studied two groups with one characterized as women who had had a diagnosis of invasive cervical cancer or CIN2 and another group randomly selected matched controls of women who did not have these diagnoses.

The team found that a specialist diagnosis of women with mental illness manifested an elevated risk of invasive cervical cancer and CIN2 but a reduced level of cervical screening involvement compared with matched controls of non-diagnosed women. Furthermore, they found that among substance misuse patients, the risk was higher for an invasive cervical cancer. On the other hand, they found the screening reduction increased for intellectual disability and autism. A higher rate of screening participation included a higher risk factor of CIN2 characterized women using prescribed psychotropic medications but there was also a documented reduced risk of invasive cervical cancer among these women as over against women with neither specialist diagnosis or medication use. The final analysis of this databased study showed that women who were suffering from a mental illness actually participate less frequently in cancer screening and also experience an elevated risk of cervical neoplasia.

Emotional adjustment to a diagnosis of cancer is a challenge to most patients regardless of the type and stage of cancer being assessed and treated. However, some cancers are more challenging than others owing to the presence of psychiatric comorbidity and the need for an active utilization of mental health care as expressed and explored by J. Keszte of the Medical Psychology Department of the University Medicine Center in Leipzig, Germany. Of particular concern for pinpointed research had to do with the aftercare treatment of laryngeal cancer surgery in relationship to psychiatric comorbidity which affects 11% of the cohort studied by the Keszte team of researchers from the Leipzig University Medical Center, the Clinical Center Dresden-Friedrichstadt, the University Hospital of Jena, the Clinical Center of Chemnitz, and the Mainz University Medical Center (Keszte, Danker, Deitz, et al., 2017). Keszte and a team of German research colleagues used a multi-centered prospective cohort study of 176 patients in an effort to assess the psychiatric comorbidity involving the utilization of various mental health services as well as psychosocial needs of laryngeal cancer patients following a partial laryngectomy (PRL) during the first year. Given the smallness of the cohort sample, the team was eager to apply an extremely refined analytical methodology to the subjects. In doing so, they devised a structured interview tool employed with patients anticipating surgery as well as an incremental assessment for 1 week, 3 months, and 1 year following the PRL.

While using standard face-to-face interview methodology, the team was particularly careful in studying psychiatric comorbidity which was assessed through the research instrument based on DSM-IV called the Structured Clinical Interview (SCID). Of the 176 cohort patients with cancer, 11% of them had a diagnosable psychiatric disorder during the first week, 15% during the third week, and 14% at the 12 month mark. Of this number 4% actually underwent psychiatric treatment or psychotherapy categorized at 2% acute, 15% emerging, and 6% chronic psychiatric comorbidity. The team found that chronically mental ill patients were characterized most commonly as younger than 65 years of age, as being female, and regularly were in need of psychological counseling. A call for more psychological counseling characterized just above a quarter of the patients in this study following one year after surgery.

Percentages were judged somewhat small regarding alcohol-related disorders for only 3% manifested alcohol-related disorders during the first week, 3% after 3 months and 8% after the 12 month period of tracking. Of this group only one patient actually received psychological treatment with another 14% expressing an unmet need for counseling with 7% calling for additional medical consultations. The disturbing reality regarding treatment protocols and modalities with such patients as these partial laryngectomy (PRL) patients was the fact that the non-treatment of any alcohol-related disorders manifested in a measurement of the cohort members indicated that this significant problem of alcohol consumption in laryngeal cancer patients constitutes a statistical reduction in quality of life and an increase in functional impairments of the patient and overall survival rates. Monitoring drinking behavior, the team argues, must continue to be a continued priority in the treatment of post-PRL patients.

Whether or not there is a real increase in the number of cancer patients being treated who also are suffering from mental illness or rather there is a great awareness of and sensitivity to the reality of mental illness present in cancer patients is not to be discussed here for, indeed, that question requires a level of sophistication the data for which either does not exist or is illusive to researchers. What is known with statistical verification is that there is being recorded now a rise in the number of reported otolaryngologic patients who are at the time of diagnosis suffering from mental illness. The sparsity of data related to the epidemiological characteristics of cancer patients being presented for otolaryngological treatment procedures who concurrently are diagnosed with a mental illness constitutes a significant arena for clinical research needed to better understand the head and neck surgery's post-operative responses to this procedure. Zaid Al-Qurayshi of the Department of Otolaryngology at the University of Iowa Hospitals and clinics in Iowa City, IA, has drawn attention to the importance of this research agenda relative to head and neck surgery and has put together a research team of oncologists and surgeons from his own hospital along with medical staff at the Tulane University School of Medicine and the Henry Ford

Health System in Detroit to focus attention upon both the presentation of this cancer by the patient and the outcomes reported in response to surgery on the part of patients suffering with a mental illness (Al-Quravshi, Rossi-Meyer, Shama, Willams, et al., 2023).

This team's research relied upon a database drawn from the Nationwide Readmissions Database from 2010 to 2015 consisting of a retrospective cross-sectional analysis of 146,182 cancer patients of which 18.3% were suffering from mental illness. What gained much research attention was the fact that there was a striking rise in the percentage of cancer patients who received otolaryngologic surgery with a history of mental illness elevating from 14.9% in 2010 to 25.0% in 2015, a significant rise in percentages which requires analysis and explanation. The team sorted out the types of mental illness affecting the otolaryngologic surgery patient. They found that the diagnoses of these patients included depression (6.9%), anxiety (5.8%), alcohol dependence (4.2%) substance dependence (2.9%), bipolar disorder (1.4%), memory disorders (1.2%), delusional disorders (0.6%), and self-harm (9.1%). This group of patients was on average above age 65, female, and subject to multiple comorbidities. Those patients with a history of mental illness were much more at risk of complications. Because clinical data has verified that cancer patients with a history of mental illness are increasingly presenting themselves for otolaryngology services and, therefore, the need to study is evidenced in this database research which has provided an epidemiological perspective calling for more systematic research by oncologists of this narrowly identifiable population.

The relationship between cognitive function, psychosocial well-being, and biomedical cancer treatment converge in the matrix of questions related to cancer and mental illness. Due to the range of cancer types coupled with the array of mental disorders to which cancer patients are susceptible, the challenge for any research team is to specify the type or types of cancer they intend to study and to identify with precision the types of psychosis or psychiatric disorders of which they are interested. Clearly all cancers and all mental illnesses cannot be studied in one venture so the specificity of type of cancer and type of mental disorder becomes the first order of business for a serious research team. A team of oncologists at the Nagoya University Graduate School of Medicine in Japan under the leadership of Satoshi Tamauchi launched an investigation precisely to scope out the nature and range of the relationship between preexisting mental disorders and the prognosis of gynecologic cancer within the context of an understanding that cancer treatment most often involves a long-term therapy protocol with follow-up monitoring where mental disorders are frequently found to affect treatment process (Tamauchi, Kajiyama, Moriyama, et al., 2019). From the Medical School's Department of Obstetrics and Gynecology, Tamauchi gathered a team of colleagues committed to this study involving 54 patients with both gynecologic cancer and mental disorders using 108 patients for a control group without mental disorders. The overall focus was on the intensity of detailed analysis rather than volume of subjects.

Because it is well-known that the treatment of cancer usually involves a long-term spell of therapy including contingent follow-up treatment and because mental disorders quite commonly have an impact upon the treatment protocol and process, this team of researchers chose to analyze cases which involved gynecologic cancer accompanied by mental disorders. Their aim was to attempt a clarification of the linkage between psychosis and the prognosis of cancer identification, assessment, and treatment. As noted earlier, 54 patients were identified for this study having gynecologic cancer accompanied by a mental disorder along with 108 control cohorts with cancer but without a mental disorder with an overall median age of 52 years. Only cancer cases in this study were used in which the patient had been diagnosed with a mental disorder prior to a diagnosis of cancer. The control patients without a mental disorder were analyzed with both groups, with and without a mental disorder (MD), adjusted for age, type of cancer, and the stage of cancer development.

The team broke the cancer patients with MD down into sub-groups of 25 schizophrenia cases, 15 depressive disorders, 4 bipolar disorders, and 10 unclassified MD patients. What somewhat amazed the research team was the fact that over the 5-year span of the study of survival rates, there was no measurable difference between cancer patients with MD and the control group without MD. However, the researchers did discover that given the advanced-stage cervical cancer patient, the prognosis proved substantially poor in light of the low rate of beginning treatment to completion. These particular patients had a measurably lower chemotherapy completion rate compared to patients with gynecologic malignancies. In the final analysis, these findings led the team to conclude that mental disorders actually do not measurably affect the prognosis of gynecologic cancers save for those with an advanced cervical cancer. They concluded, therefore, that the elevation of the quality of care for the low rate of initial treatment completion might prove to be a significantly important point of address to improve a better prognosis in advanced cervical cancer cases.

A particularly distinctive specialization in research topics for dealing with cancer and mental illness is that of a concern as to the relevance of angiogenesis in schizophrenic development in cancer patients. The topic at the time of the Lopes research team's research article was a hot topic but was more characterized by heat than light. Rui Lopes of the Faculty of Medicine of the University of Porto in Portugal was joined by several colleagues who were especially interested in the possibility that angiogenesis might constitute a missing connector between schizophrenia and cancer (Lopes, Soares, Figueiredo-Braga, Coelho, 2014). Recognizing that the formation of new blood vessels is a characteristic of both cancer and schizophrenia, this team under Lopes' leadership set about to investigate the connectivity of cancer and schizophrenia by engaging in a non-systematic review of the research published literature listed on PubMed.

Their efforts involved a summary of that current literature with an eye towards the development of a hypothesis suggesting reasons for a decrease in this relationship recorded in the data with special attention to the potential role of angiogenesis biology constituting a linked matrix of significance. They reached a general conclusion that there did exist some evidenced linked to epidemiology, genetic, molecular and biochemical studies implying an interplay between the pathophysiology of schizophrenia and angiogenesis. This research team of oncologists came to the conclusion that a concentrated effort in further analysis of angiogenesis in schizophrenia might offer more insights into links to cancer facilitating eventual cancer treatment options.

Studies of the relationship, such as it might be, between cancer and psychiatric disorders constitute a complex convergence of disparate and conflicting results. Three levels of findings have been reported in the journals such that disputed results are commonplace. One of the most striking limitations of these three levels of findings, i.e., some finding lower levels of mortality while others find no particularly valid linkage of cancer and mental illness with the overall shortcoming being that no single data base has been consistently used across the full spectra of databased studies. This challenging and baffling problem resulted in a major investigation into the value of a consistently utilized database for probing of all relevant relationship issues. It was Steve Kisley of the Department of Psychiatry at the School of Medicine at the University of Queensland (Australia) who with two other colleagues from the Princess Alexandra Hospital of Brisbane and the University of Western Australia in Perth chose specifically to address the question of why psychiatric patients have a higher rate of cancer mortality compared to the general population (Kisley, Forsyth, Lawrence, 2016). Their particular critique of current studies at the time was that these studies, as important as they proved to be, made the unfortunate mistake of not comparing incidences of cancer and mortality using the population and methodology of the same cohort such that comparisons were judged commonly to be compromised.

Kisley and team gathered data for the years 2002 to 2007 for the general Queensland population covering both mental health records and cancer registrations along with death records with the intention of comparing cancer incidence and mortality rates in psychiatric patients based on an historical cohort. Within the database of 89,992 new cancer cases, there were 3,349 individuals identified as suffering from a mental illness. Overall, they found that incidences of cancer in patients studied in this cohort were comparable to the Queensland general population for most mental illnesses but noted that rates for dementia were actually lower than the general population as well as that of schizophrenia. However, for the primary psychiatric diagnoses, they discovered that mortality rates were actually increased in psychiatric patients. The team discovered, to their surprise, that lifestyle issues such as alcohol and tobacco use were not actually relevant in identifying individuals with mental illness any more so than among the general population who were not likely to develop cancer but were more like to die from it. The need to improve cancer screening for this population became self-evident to the research team.

One of the greatest challenges in psychiatric oncology is the identification of types of mental illness relative to types of cancers. It is as impossible to speak of mental illness or psychiatric disorders as a single entity as it is to speak of cancer as a single biological phenomenon. Though early in the last century it was inevitable that such reductionist conclusions loomed in the minds of the general public as well as early researchers, but by the late 1900s the realization that refinement in the identification of cancer types was as important as the refinement of mental illness types. The emergence of the DSM reference text developed by the American Psychiatric Association tremendously accelerated the sophistication of psychiatric disorder identification and so likewise with oncology research during the same period of time. A major databased study of the relationship between prolactin breast cancer risk and antipsychotics used in the treatment of patients with schizophrenia was led by M. DeHert of the Department of Neurosciences at the KU Leuven University Psychiatric Centre in Kortenberg, Belgium, with colleagues from the University of Leicester and the University of Leuven (DeHert, Peuskens, Sabbe, et al., 2016). They began their research agenda with the presumption, based on variously gathered databased studies in a meta-analysis, that breast cancer was more likely than not more frequently detected in female patients with schizophrenia than in the general population. What has recently proven most informative in the development of experimental and epidemiological research is the discovery of the central importance of prolactin (PRL) in mammary carcinogenesis. This realization led this research team to explore further the possibility of a relationship between antipsychotic-induced hyperprolactinemia (HPRL) and the risk of breast cancer in women suffering from schizophrenia.

Using MEDLINE data gathered from the literature covering 1950 to January 2015, the research team focused on English publications of clinical trials in an attempt to locate and integrate data from the current state of knowledge relative to breast cancer risks in schizophrenic women and the probable relationship between HPRL and antipsychotic medications. They initiated this research agenda based on the reasonable assurance that a growing range of studies was beginning to strongly suggest the involvement of PRL in breast carcinogenesis in spite of the fact that studies dealing with human prospective studies were arguably limited, somewhat equivocal, and essentially correlative with risk ratios ranging from less than 2.0 for premenopausal women to just over 2.0 for postmenopausal women. Though the ratio various was minimal, it was taken seriously as suggestive of a potentially looming problem in cancer care owing partly to these various studies actually not taking full account of the local production of the PRL in breast epithelium. Furthermore, at this point in time there is still no reliable evidence that antipsychotic medication measurably contributes to an increased risk of breast malignancy and even mortality. The research team concludes that other risk factors beyond PRL may be of actual greater relevance in the development of breast cancer within the female cancer population who suffer from schizophrenia including such contributing factors as nulliparity, obesity, diabetes mellitus, and such unhealthy lifestyle factors as alcohol dependence, smoking, and low physical activity.

Clinically substantiated observations consistently validate the conclusion that psychiatric disorders and mental illness generally are not biochemically linked in patients with cancer such that any serious investigation into the nature and function of the linkage between cancer and mental illness must inevitably orient around the psychosocial spectrum of cancer (Morgan, 2023a). An outgrowth of concern regarding this matrix of information has to do with the statistically verified fact that cancer patients are more likely to die earlier than the general population if they suffering from schizophrenia. This observation is further suggestive of the psychosocial spectrum of cancer care rather than a biochemically linked etiology. Kelly E. Irwin of Massachusetts General Hospital Center for Psychiatric Oncology and Behavioral Sciences in Boston has been joined by colleagues in the MGH Schizophrenia Program to specifically address the issues related to existing disparities in the care of geriatric schizophrenic cancer patients (Irwin, Henderson, Knight, Pirl, 2014). This research team predicated its initial research agenda on the basis of a delineated disparity reflected in systems-level factors and expansive stigma regarding mental illness generally and among the elderly specifically.

Based on the national data base provided by the Center for Disease Control (CDC), this team was eager to early on point out that individuals suffering from schizophrenia have a measurably higher rate of cancer mortality than the general population and commonly have enduring medical comorbidity issues. These individuals tend to reticence in attending to routine cancer screening and frequently present a more advanced stage of cancer when they do seek medical attention. The team found that cancer patients suffering from schizophrenia were disinclined to accept chemotherapy or radiotherapy and commonly experienced complications from surgery thus accessing palliative care regularly. In spite of these patients' reluctance there did exist in most cases the opportunity for the medical, surgical, and radiation oncologists to engage the patient with an attending staff including care physicians to regularly service the receptive patient. Irwin and colleagues offered an expansive review of data available at the time dealing with overall cancer-specific mortality issues with patients suffering from schizophrenia addressing specifically a spectrum of disparities in cancer care ranging from screening, diagnosis, treatment to end-of-life treatment and care. They chose to identify specific care and treatment challenges for this classification of patient including communication, informed consent, and risk of suicide. As practitioners of oncological care, they made specific suggestions regarding treatment modalities including suggestions regarding research addressing the disparities in cancer care for patients suffering from schizophrenia. Indicating the value of patient care embodied in psychiatric oncology, they emphasized the potential for increased care and treatment of cancer patients with schizophrenia as illustrated in the clinical work of the attending medical staff.

In the past 20 years, there has been an international rise in consciousness within the oncology community of the glaring disparity between the quality of care for cancer patients based on their mental health with patients suffering from a psychiatric disorder receiving less attention than psychologically healthy cancer patients. The coming of psychiatric oncology decades before has now provided a matrix within which this disparity can more effectively be addressed. A broad spectrum of variables constitutes the arena within which research is now on an accelerated pace of development including such sub-sets as geriatric schizophrenia and the gradations of care relative to the socio-economic status of the patient. The psychosocial spectrum of cancer care embodied in the work of psychiatric oncology continues to gain international attention and respect. Ruth Cunningham of the University of Otago Wellington, NZ, along with several colleagues in social psychiatry have demonstrated the effectiveness of such a focused research project by examining a national cohort of New Zealand cancer patients (Cunningham, Sarfati, Stanley, Peterson, Collings, 2015). In a concerted effort to sort out the reasons why there is a worse cancer survival rate among patients suffering from a mental illness as compared to those with no presenting mental health issues, Cunningham and colleagues chose to study the linkage between various cancer types and a spectrum of psychiatric diagnoses. This approach constituted a significant advance in this field of cancer and mental illness research.

Drawing from the New Zealand Breast and Colorectal Cancer Registry (2006-2010), the team linked this data to psychiatric hospitalization records for adults ages 18 to 64 years old. Relying upon the Cox regression data, the team compared cancer-specific survival rates for individuals using recent psychiatric services and those who did not take advantage of such. They integrated into the study the contributions of data relative to deprivation, comorbidity, and stage at the time of diagnosis for sufferers of schizophrenia or bipolar affective disorder (classified as Group A) and the remainder of the cohort who took advantage of other mental health services (classified as Group B). This national database provided 8,762 individuals with breast cancer and 4,022 with colorectal cancer. Of the former group 440 had consulted with psychiatric services and latter 190 with psychiatric services. Confounding adjustments made by the research team showed a death risk from breast cancer increased in both Group A and Group B but only in colorectal cancer for Group A. Interestingly, late stage diagnosis was linked to survival differentials for Group A and comorbidity for both Group A and B. An anticipated but nevertheless disturbing realization illustrated that severe physical disease sufferers combined with delays in cancer diagnosis within this population with identified psychotic disorders constituted the clear causes of worse cancer survival rates in New Zealand for users of psychiatric services.

An abiding topic of research in oncology is that of the recognizable correlation between patients with cancer and that of a mental disorder, particularly schizophrenia, such that mortality statistics can more clearly reflect that relationship. Factoring in the stages of diagnosed cancer with treatment modalities and protocols when applied to in-hospital mortality issues constitutes a major issue of research for medical institutions as well as practicing oncologists. The recognition of psychiatric disorders in hospitalized cancer patients is a consistent field of databased research. Hanako Ishikawa of the Graduate School of Medicine at the University of Tokyo has initiated just such a research project assisted by his colleagues from the Medical School with the focus upon early detection, diagnosis, and treatment of cancer patients with schizophrenia (Ishikawa, Yasunaga, Matsui, Fushimi, Kawakami, 2016). A significant feature of this research initiative is that of the nature and scope of the prognosis of hospitalized cancer patients with schizophrenia as compared to such patients who did not have a diagnosed mental illness.

By accessing a nationally sponsored in-patient database maintained by the Japanese medical and government agencies, this team put together a retrospective matched-pair cohort of hospitalized patients with gastrointestinal cancer. In an effort to compare cancer stages at the time of admission, invasive treatment modalities and protocols, and exclusively designed for 30-day in-hospital mortality rates for both cancer patients with schizophrenia (n=2,495) and patients without psychiatric disorders (n=9,980), the research team employed a multivariable ordinal/binary logistic regressions model for the analysis. Ishikawa and colleagues found that of the case group being studied, these patients manifested a higher percentage of stage IV cancer with a decreased rate of invasive treatment characterized by a higher in-hospital mortality rate. The overall findings proved helpful in assessing the relationship between diagnosis and in-hospital care such that patients with both gastrointestinal cancer and schizophrenia manifested clearly a more advanced stage of cancer with a lower rate of invasive treatment and higher in-hospital mortality than patients without a mental disorder.

CHAPTER THREE

Disparities in Mental Illness Among Cancer Care Providers

Cancer Care Providers; Disparities in Treatment of the Mentally Ill; Family Issues and Social Care; Cancer Survivorship; Cancer and Mortality Rates

An enduring challenge to the oncology research community is that of understanding the complexities involved in documenting disparities in cancer care treatment. Sometimes, these disparities are easily identified and categorized on the basis of such simple variables as education, gender, geography, demographics, types of cancer, and stages of cancer development. By tracking these variables the converging reasons for disparity often become self-evident. When it comes to an international perspective on cancer screening involving patients with mental illness or psychiatric disorders, the challenge becomes rapidly more complicated. Another challenge facing international research is the availability of data sources and engaging a team of researchers from a variety of internationally respected research institutions. Once the focus of the research is set, in this case that of the disparities in cancer screening of individuals with mental illness distributed throughout the world, and the identification of internationally distinguished researchers at multiple research institutions throughout the world, then the work can begin.

Left to the editorial discrimination of *Lancet Psychiatry,* just such a winning combination of ingredients was identified thanks to the creative efforts of Marco Solmi of the Neurosciences Department of the University of Padua (Italy). Calling on a dozen internationally distinguished medical research professionals from as many research institutions representing as many countries, Solmi mobilized a team effort to explicate the disparities in cancer screening practices involving patients with mental illness from throughout the world totaling a sampling of individuals numbering 4,717,839 (501,599 patients with mental illness and 4,216,280 serving as a control group) (Solmi, Firth, Miola, Fornaro, et al., 2020). The presenting problem for this research team was the fact that cancer patients suffering from mental illness have a much higher mortality rate than the general cancer population. Does this particular class of patient receive less cancer screening than the general population and, if so, is this a contributing factor to mortality?

The thoroughness of this databased study is impressive by any international standard and, therefore, must be considered one of the most important studies of its kind at the time of execution. Using meta-analysis, this team systematically reviewed PubMed and PsycINFO with no language limitations placed on the published documents with all references physically verified by hand from the inception of the study through to May 5, 2019. The review of the literature covered all types of cancer screening of mentally ill cancer patients. The odds ratio (OR) of cancer screening in patients with mental illness compared to the general population constituted the primary outcome and using the Newcastle-Ottawa Scale, an assessment for quality validated the heterogeneity of the data resulting in this study being registered with PROSPERO, CRD42018114781 (authenticity of data sources).

The sampling of 4,717,839 individuals (501,599 patients with mental illness and 4,216,280 serving as a control group) was drawn from 47 publications of which nearly 70% were involved in screening for breast cancer (296,699 individuals with mental illness), cervical cancer (688 with mental illness), colorectal cancer (153,283 with mental illness), lung and gastric cancer (420 with mental illness), ovarian cancer (37 with mental illness), and prostate cancer (803 with mental illness). Throughout this study, the research team found that cancer screening generally was substantially less frequent in cancer patients with any type of mental illness as compared to the general population and though this was anticipated the size of the data proved conclusively validating of this expectation. What proved most disturbing to the medical community globally was the discovery (as anticipated) that even though there was the recognition of the increasing mortality rate from cancer among patients suffering a mental illness, this particular grouping of patient types consistently and globally received a reduced level of cancer screening and particularly among women with schizophrenia.

In terms of medical history and its relationship to cancer research, there is a plethora of medical and biological researchers who are given credit for advancing the scientific study of cell division relative to cancer. Rudolf Virchow must be cited at the head of this list for in the mid- 1800s his research led to an understanding of what became cellular pathology in which he discovered that every cell stems from another cell and, thus, the launching of what eventuated into oncological research. The plethora of specializations in cancer research today constitutes a legion of discoveries and oncology is now elevated to a leading medical science field in the world. Some applications of cancer research have concentrated on types of cancer such as lung, breast, and prostate while others have focused on the relevance of age and social status and even education. Sung Jin Park has created a research team addressing the fundamental issues related to the relationship between severe mental illness and socio-economics status of cancer patients and their treatment and survival rates in developing countries. From the Institute of Psychiatry at King's College London, Sung Jin Park brought together a team of medical researchers interested in this topic representing a variety of distinguished institutions including the Amrita Institute of Medical Sciences and Research Centre in Kochi, India, the Hamad Medical Corporation in Qatar, and the National Health Science Foundation Trust in London (Park, Wai, Pavithran, Kunheir, Valsrai, 2021).

The challenge and focus of this team's research efforts centered around the issue of inequities of treatment of patients suffering from severe mental illness and the resulting rise in mortality among cancer patients in developing countries (aka low and middle income countries). One of the precipitating motivations for this team's efforts arose from the data suggested in the research literature that responsible studies have been done on high-income countries regarding cancer patients and serious mental illness treatments and survival rates but a virtual research desert exists for developing countries. It was Park and team's intent to focus international attention to this disparity of treatment among developing countries when it comes to the care and survival of cancer patients suffering from severe mental illness. They particularly wished to elevate the relevance of integrating psycho-oncological care of severe mental illness patients suffering from cancer in an effort to contribute to a reduction of blatant disparities and inequities in this field linked to socio-economic factors. In order to conduct an initial literature search and review, the team consulted two internationally respected databases, viz., PubMed and Google Scholar, in which 80 research articles were actually identified and used in this study. The effectiveness of a literature search is tied to the scope of the search words used. These words were carefully selected keywords including severe mental illness, SMI, schizophrenia, bipolar disorder, cancer, low to middle-income countries, low and middle-income countries, psycho-oncology, HPV vaccine, cancer incidence, cancer mortality, cancer control, cancer screening, cancer treatment and palliative care.

Based on this analysis, the team concluded that due to such variables as social, psychological, economical and healthcare issues, there was documented an elevated rate of cancer in both low and middle income countries as well as a rise in the number of cancer patients suffering from serious mental illness in developing countries, i.e., low and middle income. There was a call for developing countries to address this issue and to elevate their resources to mitigate the on-going disparity in cancer care.

As with mental illness a patient's response to a surgical intervention can be a challenging prospect of adjustment. Of course, the operative variables affecting both mental illness and cancer surgery is linked to the type of mental illness or psychiatric disorder and the type of cancer surgery to which the patient is subjected and then called upon to respond with hope. Studies have consistently shown that a cancer patient suffering from a mental illness is greatly challenged to maintain a stable attitude and response to the diagnosis and treatment of the disorder. The same is certainly true of a cancer diagnosis leading to serious surgical procedures and the necessity of responding with confidence towards the future. One of the most demanding and complex relationships in this matrix of health care is that of the female patient undergoing a surgical procedures for mastectomy for breast cancer who concurrently is suffering from a severe mental illness (aka in this study as a Severe Persistent Mental Illness SPMI). Such a confluence of demanding health situations constitutes a major area of needed research which Anagha J. Deshpande of the Alix School of Medicine's Mayo Clinic in Scottsdale, AZ, launched. In a concerted effort to examine the complex relationship between a patient's severe mental illness undergoing surgery for breast cancer, Deshpande put together a research team of oncologists and psychiatrists from the Mayo Clinics in Scottsdale, AZ, Rochester, MN, and Jacksonville, FL to tackle this bafflingly convoluted linkage of mental illness and cancer surgery (Deshpande, Bhandarkar, Bobo, Bydon, Niazi, McLaughlin, 2023). Since most outcomes of cancer patients suffering from a mental illness consistently prove to be less than satisfactory, this research team chose to specifically focus on to what extent there is a profoundly serious devolution of survival outcome from breast cancer of patients with a mental illness.

Drawing their data from the National Inpatient Sample (2016-2018), they were able to identify 670 patients with both breast cancer and a severe mental illness through the use of propensity score matching. This was followed by the use of multivariate analysis, Kruskal-Wallis tests, and conditional logistic regression in which they were able to compare the demographics of this group and the documented outcomes. Of the 670 cancer patients studied (536 without a serious mental illness and 134 with), the team found that patients with a severe persistent mental illness were linked with bilateral mastectomy with a decreased frequency of breast reconstruction while these patients were clearly linked to a more extended hospitalization accompanied by an increased risk of developing a post-procedural infection as well as sepsis. The team was able to formalize their conclusions regarding this database by pointing out that SPMI was linked to bilateral mastectomy, more extended hospital stays, and an increased risk for post-procedural infection and sepsis which led them to emphasize the need for a more robust elevated use of standardized screening methods which have proven effective in identifying SPMI in cancer patients with breast cancer.

A particularly troubling characteristic of cancer patients suffering from a mental illness is the fact that the life expectancy of these patients is 15 to 20 years shorter than that of the general population. Mortality issues have always constituted a primary research area for oncologists and there are cancers with a morbidity rate spread across a broad spectrum of possible longevities with some being extremely short while others fall within the scope of a Long-Term Condition (LTC). However, it falls to the cancer patient suffering from a psychiatric disorder to face the briefest mortality rate across the global spectrum. Still there is much research needed to be done to address this reality with treatment protocols designed specifically to address this mortality rate. There are but two ways of moving forward with this search for answers and that is with both clinical databased research and with consistent and sustained assessment of scholarly literature published in the medical journals of findings from researchers around the world. Laura Charlesworth of the Sheffield Hallman University's College of Health, Wellbeing and Life Sciences in the United Kingdom has been joined by Colette Fegan and Russell Ashmore of that University's faculty to address this issue through a carefully executed scoping review of the published literature in the medical journals. The parameters of the literature research project focused on to what extent and how a severe mental illness in a cancer patient impacts the mortality outcome (Charlesworth, Fegan, Ashmore, et al., 2023).

This research team began with the statistically validated fact that an individual with a severe mental illness has a 15 to 20 years shorter longevity than the general population. When patients suffering from a severe mental illness are also diagnosed with cancer their life expectancy is shorter than cancer patients without a psychiatric disorder. Charlesworth and colleagues chose to investigate through a scoping review recently published databased research in the journals the impact on cancer outcomes where individuals have been diagnosed with a pre-existing SMI. Their literature search was expansive in that it covered all English published articles between 2001 and 2021 gathered from PsychINFO, PubMed, PsycArticles and the Cochrane Librar. They restricted their article assessment to only those which were published after a peer review. Based on both the presenting title of the article and an abstract screening process, the team followed this procedure with a full text analysis of selected articles dealing with the impact of severe mental illness on cancer covering these central issues including stage of cancer at the time of the diagnosis, survival rates, treatment access and quality of life for the cancer patient. Out of 1,226 articles found, 27 actually met the criteria set by the team for analysis but disappointingly there was no single article which met the selection criteria which dealt precisely with the perspective of the treatment patient nor did any article deal specifically with the impact of a severe mental illness in a cancer patient had upon the patient's quality of life. From these selected articles, however, the researchers identified three topical areas produced by the article assessments, viz., cancer related mortality, stage of diagnosis, and access to state appropriate treatment.

In the absence of a large-scale cohort study and, therefore, relying on a literature review the study of populations with comorbidity involving both severe mental illness and a cancer diagnosis constitutes a monumental challenge to analysis. Relying, then, upon a coping review characterized by heterogeneous data presenting diagnoses of both SMI and cancer, this collection of assessed review articles suggested that cancer is clearly related to mortality which is inevitably increased in the general population of individuals with a pre-existing severe mental illness (SMI). Also, cancer patients with an SMI are more susceptible to a metastatic disease at the point of diagnosis but less likely to actually receive appropriate treatment for the presenting stage of cancer. Clearly demonstrated by this research team in their assessment of this expansive range of published research is the fact that patients with a pre-existing severe mental illness with a cancer diagnosis are much more likely to have a specific mortality rating far below the general population. They suggested the complexities of the issues related to the comorbidity of SMI and cancer result often in the patient receiving less optimal treatments for both illnesses characterized by common interruptions to regular treatment protocols as well as frequent delays in the treatment regimen itself.

In spite of the expansive and accelerated evidence of the efficacy of oncologists and cancer centers addressing the psychosocial spectrum of cancer care, there continues to be a vacuum in databased studies of health care workers including oncologists and psychiatrists actively engaged in a robust referral protocol for cancer patients suffering from mental illness. In order to move forward with a more responsive awareness of the efficacy of emotional care of these patients, there needs to be both the recognition of the personal, professional, and institutional barriers to referral protocol and accountability. Under the leadership of Moritz Philipp Gunther of the Department of Consultation-Liaison-Psychiatry and Psychosomatic Medicine at the University Hospital of Zurich, Switzerland, Gunther has put together a team of medical professionals from both the University Hospital of Zurich as well as the Department of Medical Psychology and Medical Sociology at the University Medical Center in Leipzig, Germany, with the specific aim of unravelling the complexities of these barriers affecting the benefits of distress screening and psychological support and referrals.

Mental disorders, length of hospitalization, and psychopharmacology are all linked to this issue of barrier identification owing to the painful fact that to-date there is little substantive research and publishing on rates of distress screening and systemic protocols for referrals of patients in psychological support. This is in spite of the fact that the evidence is clear that emotional distress is common among cancer patients and particularly among those patients suffering from a mental disorder. The need for a mandatory component of best-practice cancer care is, according to Gunther and team, crucial for the elevation of the quality of care for cancer patients in mental distress. For their research method protocol, they used latent class analysis (LCA) to select homogeneous subgroups from among the 4,837 patients who had been diagnosed with cancer between 2011 and 2019. In this analysis, there were four subgroups selected according to characteristic parameters such that patients manifesting a diagnosable mental disorder as well as utilization of psychopharmacology constituted the smallest number of patients actually submitting to screening for distress. This same group of male patients who were 65 years old and older was less likely to submit to offers of psychological support but patients who experienced hospitalization for 28 days or more were predictably most inclined to receive and benefit from both screening and the reception of psychological support.

Based on these findings, the research team encouraged the clinical and researcher staff not to overlook the emotional needs of the cancer patient with a mental disorder and to implement psychopharmacological treatment protocols particularly for male patients and elderly patients by providing a more robust screening for distress and increased access to psychological services.

A fundamental and essential characteristic of science is the absolute necessity of consultation and collaboration within the scientific community. A particularly meaningful instance of this feature is within the medical sciences for little has been accomplished without the convergence of knowledge and insights gained from a broad spectrum of research from a wide range of clinical perspectives. The emergence of the field of oncology itself has been built upon the foundation blocks of cellular biology and biochemistry applied to the study of a particular somatic disease, i.e., cancer. Growing out of this monumental development of oncology has emerged a broad spectrum of specializations and in recent years there has been the gradual recognition that the emotional side of cancer care has a rightful place at the table of cancer care research. Psychiatric oncology has developed under the initial leadership of Dr. Jimmie Holland of the Sloan-Kettering Cancer Institute in New York and the inevitable appearance of a professional body of psychiatric oncologists (aka psychooncology) has led to the publication of an internationally distinguished research medical journal addressing specifically the psychosocial spectrum of cancer care. Under the leadership of Luigi Grassi of the University of Ferrara and with the collaboration of Michelle B. Riba of the University Hospital Psychiatric Unit of S. Anna Hospital in Italy, a composite survey of research in this specialization taken from eight different countries has been compiled in an issue of *Psychooncology* to address the topic of disparities and inequalities in cancer care of patients with severe mental illness (Grassi, Riba (2021).

Thanks to this energetic sub-field of specialization in oncological research, there is now the universal recognition that cancer patients suffering from severe mental illness are most commonly at an extreme risk of stigmatization such that poor quality of physical care accompanies the overall somatic state of health. A higher rate of morbidity including a diminished prognosis of comorbidity is well above the general population's longevity prospects for cancer patients with a severe mental illness have a likelihood of a reduced life expectancy of from 10 to 20 years. In recognition of these disparities and inequities in the medical treatment of cancer patients with severe mental illness, the Editorial Board of *Psychooncology* took the initiative under the oversight of Grassi and Riba to launch a special issue of that journal addressing precisely these disparities intending to examine three specific areas. They include mortality due to cancer, difficulties involved in communication systems between oncology and psychiatric teams and the clearly established need for a more systematic structuring of issues related to intervention including screening, prevention, and treatment. A presenting concern by these researchers was the persistent misunderstanding and stigmatized diminishment of cancer care provided for patients suffering from a severe mental illness. Researchers from eight countries contributed to this collection of published scholarship focusing on the fundamental blocks in patient care related to the patients themselves and clinical and institutional problems of service and understanding commonly resulting in fragmented and disjointed systems of sustained care. These published papers validated the data showing that cancer patients with severe mental illness consistently experience an elevated rate of mortality compared to the general population easily attributed to a misunderstanding or faulty misperception of the nature of this class of patient.

Growing out of this monumentally important collaboration of research authors were an array of conclusions leading to specific and practical recommendations by these authors. The overall improvement of care for this class of patient included, for example, the need for specifically developed guidelines and fundamental clinical protocols developed with the cancer patient suffering from a severe mental illness for implementation in a mental healthcare setting. They called for an aggressively broad base of databased research addressing these disparities, and an elevated vision of psychiatric oncology as the essential ingredient in the collaborative work of oncologists and psychiatrists working with cancer patients suffering from mental illness.

The range of issues related to the on-going disparities and equities of treatment for cancer patients with mental illness is substantial. However, there are still areas where more databased studies might prove helpful in collapsing the quality care gap between the non-mentally ill cancer patient and the patient suffering from a psychiatric disorder. Though the Americans have been engaged in following this relationship for some time, it appears that the British have not kept pace such that in the United Kingdom. There seems to be a shortage of databased studies in the UK investigating the relationship of breast cancer screening uptake and women who also are suffering from a mental illness. This is particularly significant for breast cancer screening uptake owing to the fact that in the UK health care is provided by the National Health Service for all women who seek coverage. A study launched by Emma Ross of the Centre for Public Health at Queen's University in Belfast included colleagues from both the Centre and the Public Health Agency of Northern Ireland drawing data from a population-based examination of the linkage of mental illness measured by the uptake of psychotropic medications on this particular category of patient (Ross, Maguire, Mairs, Hall, Donnelly, O'Reilly, et al., 2021).

The breadth of this national databased study was impressive as some 57,328 patient cohort of women suffering from both breast cancer and mental illness identified by the 2011 Census of the Northern Ireland Longitudinal Study. These patients followed through a single 3-year screening cycle (2011-2014) as recorded by the National Health Service Breast Screening Programme. This study identified mental illness using a receipt of psychotropic medication taken during the 3 months immediately preceding the screening event with the Census records providing information for both individual and household-level characteristics. The whole study was conducted in 2019. Members in this cohort had actually received no more than one prescription for psychotropic medication in the 3 months immediately preceding the screening invitation. Actual participating attendance was reduced by 15% and proved particularly low for women who had been prescribed antipsychotics, anxiolytics, and hypnotics.

Based on these findings, the team was able to report that there was evidence of a substantial disparity in breast cancer screening uptake for those women suffering from mental illness such that the researchers suggested that the focusing of medical intervention is especially called for in this cohort of women in an attempt to reduce avoidable breast cancer mortality. This call was noted urgently owing to the prevalence and increasing rise of mental illness among women with breast cancer.

A particularly distinguishing international characteristic of this particular scientific enterprise is both the range of research topics falling within its purview and the ready willingness to share findings of a significant nature with the scientific community through publication. Any topic of research significance eventually finds itself discussed and researched collaboratively through the printed and internet media such that no subject of any real importance is ever perpetually overlooked. Beyond empirical studies of gathered data through international networks, another approach to topical research is through literary analysis such that any significant topic relevant within the scientific community finds itself inevitably written about in the scholarly journals. One such topic which is gaining more attention than in previous decades is that of the relevance of the socioeconomic demographics relative to a particular type of cancer comparing countries of high versus low and medium income levels as a telling variable in assessing the quality of care of its citizenry.

The relationship between cancer and mental illness constitutes one of the major fields of robust research. Zoe J. Walker of the Department of Psychiatry at the University of Toronto has put together a team of researchers from her university along with a member of the Royal Hobart Hospital in Australia specifically inquiring into the issue of cancer patients suffering from depression, anxiety, and other mental disorders in low and lower-middle income countries (aka developing countries) as reported in the scholarly literature (Walker, Xue, Jones, Ravindran ,2021). Whether or not and to what extent poverty is linked causally to the development of cancer is not the question here in Walker's team research but what is the driving force of their inquiry is the documented fact that cancer is a rising public health issue in low and middle income countries though the research on this trend has yet to be thoroughly examined according to the Human Development Index (HDI). Walther and colleagues set out to actually examine systematically the presence of research literature addressing this phenomenon particularly regarding the prevalence, professional involvement, and actual treatment protocols for cancer patients suffering from a mental illness within these developing countries (LLMICs).

They set about their search of scholarly publications by systematically examining the aggregated information provided by Medline, PsycINFO, EMBASE, and CINAHL. Using the approach called a Random Effects Meta-Analysis (REMA), they sought to identify the collection of articles dealing with the prevalence of significant depression and anxiety disorders within this specific population as defined by the *Diagnostic and Statistical Manual of Mental Disorders* (DSM-5) and by the *International Classification of Diseases* (ICD). The actual prevalence of depression and anxiety qualitatively reflected in the reviewed published literature identified these disorders based on self-report tools as well as the prevalence of other unspecified mental disorders. This included associated factors of depressive and anxiety symptoms with special attention to the identification and delineation of the actual treatment protocols for mental illness embraced in these developing countries. The range and depth of this literature search was impressive for covering a 15 year span of time there were some 40 specifically published studies examined. The collected prevalence of these disorders being examined was within the definitional parameters set by the DMS-5 and the ICD such that 21% of these articles reflected major depression and anxiety disorders with symptoms for such most commonly associated with both an advanced disease and a lower level of education among the patient population. An aside was the examination of four studies which evaluated treatment options to the served population which included three for psychotherapy effectiveness and one evaluating a yoga program.

In the final analysis and to no one's surprise, the prevalence of depression and anxiety within the cancer population was measurably higher in the LLMICs than what was commonly found in upper-income (developed) countries demonstrating a general characterization of a significantly underappreciated disease burden on the LLMICs population. The team, therefore, suggested that cancer health care workers and clinicians be encouraged to maintain or develop a robust approach to psychiatric symptomatology with the notion that such a response from the service personnel and institutions would greatly improve the quality of life among the population of developing societies and reduce both morbidity and mortality over time.

Cancer screening and early detection has its own checkered history of development and adoption within the medical community. As early as the 1920s, there was a movement to introduce screening for Pap test by oncologists who first applied this new procedure to cervical cancer. Though initially the medical community was reluctant to embrace this new approach, not an uncommon characteristics of the traditionalism in medical practice, following the American Cancer Society's endorsement of the test during the 1960s. Screening has now become commonplace though not universally available or applied and not available to all cancer patients relative to their socioeconomic status, nationality, and particularly their mental health. Since the introduction of screening for cervical cancer, for example, the mortality rate has dropped 50% in the United States but even today it is more than two and half times likely in the United Kingdom that cancer patients die prematurely who are suffering from severe mental illness. Robert Stephen Kerrison of the School of Health Sciences at the University of Surrey in England put together an oncology research team of medical professionals for the specific purpose of investigating the inequalities in cancer screening participation comparing adult cancer patients with mental illness to those without mental illness based on a cross-sectional analysis of primary care data based on the English Screening Programme. Because of the disparities involved, Kerrison and colleagues sought to determine if and to what extent low participation in the screening program is a contributing factor to mortality in the UK.

The database for the Kerrison team study was massive drawn from the Clinical Practice Research Datalink identifying cancer patients with a severe mental illness participating in a bowel cancer screening (1.71 million adults), breast cancer screening (1.34 million adults), and cervical cancer screening (2.5 million). They used a multivariate logistic regression method of data analysis in an attempt to identify a possible linkage between a serious mental illness and screening participation. What the team found was that the actual cancer screening participation among this large database was lower among the adults with severe mental illness than those who did not suffer from a SMI but screening participation was lowest among those cancer patients suffering from schizophrenia followed by other psychoses and finally bipolar disorder. Participation registered lowest among patients with a SMI who resided in the most deprived areas of the country and particularly with Black ethnicity.

The conclusion to this databased study led the team to point out that cancer screening participation proves lowest among patients with an SMI with ethnicity playing a negative role as well as socioeconomic standing in deprived areas which showed serious mental illness to the highest in the population.

In the face of on-going challenges and opportunities for advancement in the understanding and treatment of a full range of cancers and likewise with the developing insights into the nature and structure of mental illness, there is a monumental challenge facing both the medical community and that of the legislative bodies of all countries when it comes to the actual expense of providing care to the sick. Disparities and inequities of all kinds affect the quality of care and the survival rates of cancer patients as well as those who have comorbidity such as mental illness. The stark reality of such disparities is seen in the use of medical care based on the cancer patient's mental acuity. The elephant in the room is the reality of the medical expense burdening the quality of care provided by hospitals and professional staff responsible for the fair distribution of assessment and treatment of all patients. The Taiwanese oncologist Jai-Jie Ma at the Department of Public Health in the China Medical University of Taichung, Taiwan, has ventured to put together a distinguished team of medical professionals to pursue a deeper and broader understanding of the disparities so blatant in the medical expenditures for cancer patients suffering from a comorbid mental disorder with an eye towards a better grasp of the relevance and efficacy of diagnosis sequence ordering protocol (Ma, Su, Mie, Chung, et al., 2023).

Because cancer constitutes the leading cause of death within Taiwan and given that the medical expenses relative to the care and treatment of cancer in Taiwan constitutes 44.8% of all other major illnesses combined reflected in insurance claims, it seems appropriate for this Taiwanese research team to address the issues surrounding the relevance of diagnosis sequence ordering to the disparities experienced in the medical care delivery system of that country. Based on the medical records available to this research team, they initially discovered that the combination of cancer and a concurrent mental disorder on the part of the patient was linked directly to the elevation of the staffing and financial medical burden of care and treatment. Through their analysis of the medical records of treatment and expenses involved in the care of cancer patients with a mental illness, they discovered that this particular category of patient requires commonly upwards of 50% more annual costs than other categories of patients. Though this category of cancer patient with mental illness has been studied throughout the system, what has not been thoroughly examined are the effects of morbidity sequence order affecting patient costs. Ma and colleagues set about to investigate medical records reporting a linkage between expenditures and comorbidity of cancer and mental illness with special focus on the impact of diagnosis sequence order.

Access to a massive governmentally developed database provided by the Ministry of Health and Welfare Data Science Center covered in this study between 2005 and 2015 involved a population-based retrospective matched cohort retrieving patients with both cancer and mental illness 20 years of age and older. The total cohort was 321,045 patients who were then divided into groups of one disease or both diseases (cancer and mental illness) including the sequence of mental disorder and cancer diagnosis. The team used a Propensity Score Matching ratio of 1:1 to pair patients with participants who were free of both diseases (cancer and mental disorders). Then, they used an Annual Cost per Patient Linear Model to actually assess the average cost of annual treatment factoring in socio-demographic and clinical variables. To track and control for the risk of high-utilization on the part of the participants, the team used a Binomial Logistic Regression as the evaluation tool.

A disturbing and enlightening finding from this study were numerous and the first tellingly informative discovery was that the "cancer only" group of participants manifested an elevated adjusted mean annual costs which was more than 5 times that of the reference group. Then, they found that by excluding patients with no cancer and including cancer patients of a diagnosis sequence order who also suffered from a mental disorder, the post-cancer mental disorder participants registered the highest expenditures coming to over 13% higher than patients diagnosed with only cancer and no mental illness. On the other hand, whereas cancer patients with any documented pre-existing mental disorder actually incurred reduced expenditures than those with cancer only. The elevated utilization of cancer care proved consistently to be a point of concern for not only were patients who were diagnosed with a post-cancer mental disorder registered a high utilization but also patients with other covariates linked to high-utilization of medical care also showed elevated utilizations among female, middle to old age, and late stage cancer.

The correlation between costs and utilization is self-evident but the identification of factors affecting both costs and utilization behavior constituted the fundamental driving force of this major study. The research team found that where mental illness is present prior to a cancer diagnosis there was a reduced effect on the utilization by patients of medical care and treatment. This they suggested might be related to the practice by the patient of a low medical compliance or even adherence in patients suffering from a mental disorder following the initial treatments after the cancer diagnosis. What was expected and confirmed by the data was that patients who developed post-cancer mental illness actually manifested the highest elevation of average annual cost of treatment expense as well as a similar result where the odds of reaching an elevated utilization status also occurred. The team's concluding suggestion was that the follow-up of cancer patient treatment suffering also from a pre-existing mental disorder might call for a greater emphasis on the fair and equitable distribution of medical resources.

Medical practitioners in the field of oncology have recognized from the beginning of the profession the fundamentally important ingredient in care of the cancer patient is the family unit and social matrix within which the patient has to deal with a diagnosis. Combine that with the common reality that cancer patients also suffer from comorbidities including a full range of psychiatric disorders within the context of the family social network and accompanying care givers. Psychiatric oncology has in the last few decades emerged as a leading theme of research addressing a full range of psychosocial spectra of cancer care issues, findings relevant to both understanding the nature and function of the family social unit as well as the central importance of the professional community's role in patient nurture. Rosangela Cruso in the Institute of Psychiatry at the University of Ferrara's Department of Biomedical and Surgical Sciences has taken the initiative to put together a research team of oncologists at her own University joined by members of the Department of Psychiatry at the University of Michigan to address specifically the challenge presented by psychosocial morbidity in the cancer patient related to family issues (Caruso, Nanni, Riba, Sabato, Grassi, 2017).

Even when developmental stages of cancer as well as the types of cancer involved are taken into consideration, there is the statistical realization that cancer is on the rise generally and that cancer patients with psychiatric disorders is keeping pace if not exceeding this reality. Both psychiatric illness such as adjustment disorders, anxiety, and depressive disorders along with neuropsychiatric disorders such as cognitive disorders subsequent to treatment and delirium have consistently registered a 30-35% reality among cancer patients. Added to this reality is the fact that such psychosocial syndromes as demoralization, health anxiety, and irritable mood syndrome are increasingly affecting the diagnostic and treatment protocols of cancer patients within the context of family life issues. Psychological distress and emotional anxieties permeate the family social unit while also being conscious of the impact that family life-style issues have upon the scope and nature of the cancer care provided by the professional team, integrating the patient's family within a consultative configuration with the medical team of cancer care givers has proven monumentally helpful in the overall well-being of the patient when it comes to both assessment and treatment protocol. This particular constellation of convergent factors affecting the patient's sustained care constituted the fundamental research agenda of Caruso and team.

One of the most challenging topics within oncology research has to do with the issues related to survivorship, i.e., individuals who have successfully survived a bout with cancer and lived to tell about it. A baffling problematic has to do with the definition of "survivor" for issues such as length of time from inception to curative state (however that is defined) and to what extent what is defined as survivorship actually characterizes the patient in question all constitute a matrix of discussion, conflict, and confusion. A further complicating factor is that of the age of the individual when cancer was first diagnosed and at what point cancer is no longer evident in the patient. Within this confluence of factors, Sapna Kaul of the University of Texas Medical Branch in Galveston, Texas, put together a team of colleagues from a variety of research institutions, viz., Baylor College of Medicine, University of Utah, and the MD Anderson Cancer Center to address fundamental issues related to the prevalence of mental distress experienced by Adolescent and Young Adult (AYA) cancer survivors and to determine what relevant correlates there might be based on data provided by the National Health Interview Survey (Kaul, Avila, Mutambudzi, Rusell, Kirchhoff, Schwartz, 2017).

In consultation with the National Health Interview Surveys, the team was provided access to a data base for 20013 and 2014 covering 875 AYA cancer survivors ages 15 to 39 years who had at least 5 years from their initial diagnosis. As a measuring tool, a comparison group was also created by the research team. Using the Kessler nonspecific mental/psychological distress scale, the researchers examined none/low, moderate, and severe distress levels among the AYA cohort. A particularly insightful component of this study had to do with whether or not the individuals being studied had actually spoken to a mental health professional within the immediately preceding year and, if so, did these individuals who were able to finance mental health care receive such an examination. The 2 groups (Group One and Group Two) were sorted using the multinomial logistic regression instrument in identifying variables relevant to the study such as demographics, smoking and alcohol behaviors, comorbidity, and actually validated mental health visits.

Of the two groups being studied in comparison, cancer survivors Group One were documented as having more mental distress and more frequently than comparison Group Two of non-cancer AYA individuals. Members of Group One, the cancer survivors, acknowledged their consistent inability to afford mental health care more frequently than members of Group Two. Furthermore, up to 75% of Group One had not spoken with a mental health professional during the entire time. In contrast, however, to Group Two, members of Group One who were continual smokers reported instances of severe distress well above that experienced by members of Group Two. Descriptive factors affecting a higher level of distress among Group One cancer survivors were such issues as either having public or no insurance coverage compared to private insurance and documented sleep-related troubles characterized Group One as well.

In their concluding remarks drawn from this databased study, the research team was quick to point out that even though AYA cancer survivors consistently report greater mental distress than non-cancer individuals, the team did emphasize that few of the Group One individuals actually received reportable mental health services leading them to conclude that clearly AYA cancer survivors are in much more need of both access to mental health screening as well as counseling as compared to non-cancer individuals if the gap between Group One and Group Two is to be closed.

The rightful focus of oncology research is the care and treatment of cancer and the cancer patient. The complexities of cancer research is complimented by the complex issues involved in the person who is the cancer patient and the coming of psychiatric oncology has proven to be a real supportive companion to clinical cancer research. The biochemical and molecular nature of cancer is complimented by the psychosocial character of the patient with the cancer. Much research of the interrelationship between the person and cancer has elevated the care and treatment of cancer patients. An emerging sub-field of psychiatric oncology is that of patient survival following the curative treatments which proved beneficial and successful in postponing mortality. However, in spite of the great deal of research on cancer itself and on the care and treatment of the patient, there has been less emphasis on the study of the cancer patient who survives including the emotional and physical ramifications of a post-cancer life. Julie A. Kittel of the University of Rochester School of Medicine in New York has put together a team of medical and psychiatric professionals from within the University of Rochester to specifically address issues related to the on-going mental health needs of the cancer patient following successful curative treatment (Kittel, Seplaki, Wijngaarden, Richman, et al., 2023).

The naïve misjudgment by the general public of a cancer patient who has been cleared of cancer and thus responded well to the curative treatment is that the issue of cancer is now "done and dusted" such that nothing more needs to be said or done! To the trained health care professional working in the field of oncology, this is far from a correct and even fair assessment. Kittel and colleagues are fully aware of the complex issues related to on-going physical and mental health challenges faced by post-cancer patients following successful treatment.

Nevertheless, there has been a sparsity of databased studies examining the on-going well-being of the cancer survivor who has responded well to curative treatment but now faces the demands of a transition from patient to an active member of society as a "cured" cancer survivor. The emotional movement by the patient from a treatment matrix to a survivor matrix is not an inconsequentially significant transition particularly during the first year following successful treatment as a post-cancer survivor. Among other concerns is the tendency on the part of some cancer patients to continue to maintain a self-image and lifestyle as a cancer patient even following an all clear assessment to a survivor status. This and other emotional issues constitute areas of important research and the Kittel team set about the identification and delineate of these complex issues. *(If and when might the cancer return is an ever present and enduring point of concern on the part of the cancer survivor and anticipatory-anxiety can become a debilitating factor.)*

Employing the medical records of 120 cancer survivors' data regarding cancer type and treatment, the research team assessed a broad spectrum of types of cancer but also personal and emotional behavioral factors including depression, anxiety, death ideation, alcohol and substance use, and demographic characteristics. Once the types of cancer treatment were identified and the patients involved in the study were given the all-clear in terms of survivor status, the team sorted out the responses of these 120 cancer survivors based on percentages such that 15% of the respondents, for example, suffered from continuing depressive symptoms as well as 15% reporting anxiety symptoms during the immediately preceding two weeks. Furthermore, 10% of the sample reported experiencing death ideation following the termination of treatment with 7.5% of those respondents reporting this on-going experience during the immediately preceding two weeks. The research team also found that younger age respondents who had suffered from a previous psychiatric diagnosis who continued a substance use were linked to depressive symptoms, anxiety symptoms, and death ideation.

The Kittel research team were able to document the common phenomenon of an elevation of depressive symptoms, anxiety symptoms, and death ideation in the cancer survivors when once given the all-clear following successful curative treatment. The team was able to determined that especially during the first year of a patient's survivorship there is a particular danger of developing mental health issues among the younger cancer survivors as well as those with a previous psychiatric diagnosis. There resulted from this study a call for a more robust study by both oncologists and primary care providers to pay close attention to modifiable risk factors among survivors of cancer for such emotional issues as depression, anxiety, and death ideation as these patients attempt a successful transition out of curative treatment and into a life without cancer treatment (and without the stigma of being labeled a cancer patient by family, friends, and society). Improving and facilitating this transition must constitutes a major area of on-going research.

A Johns Hopkins School of Medicine team commenced a databased study stating the fact that cancer is the second leading cause of death among cancer patients with serious mental illness and that these same patients received a disproportionately lower rate of screening than other cancer patients without mental illness. Karly A. Murphy and a research team of medical professionals from Johns Hopkins School of Medicine set out to examine a litany of possible predictors of cancer screening among a population insured by

Medicaid for both Black and White enrollees who had a documented record of a serious mental illness (Murphy, Daumit, McGinty, et al., 2021). The focus was on a data base provided by the State of Maryland's Medicaid program covering cancer patients suffering from a mental illness (most commonly schizophrenia and bipolar disorder) and categorized by ethnicity which has already been validated as a link to the differentiation rate of cancer screening. What factors affect the rate of cancer screening among this classification of cancer patient, namely, Black and White Medicaid covered cancer patients, granted that this classification of patient registers a utilization rate of cancer screening far below the general population.

Based on the enrollment eligibility of Black and White participants in the Maryland Medicaid administrative claims data, this research team studies 40,622 cervical cancer patients, 9,818 breast cancer patients, 19,306 colorectal cancer patients, and 4,887 prostate cancer patients. Besides examining the socio-demographic levels of each individual, the clinical factors considered included what was designated co-occurring substance use disorder, medical comorbidities, psychiatric diagnosis, and obstetric-gynecologic and primary care utilization. They also factored county-level characteristics such as metropolitan status, mean household income, and primary care workforce capacity. All of this data was linked with cancer screening by employing a generalized estimating equation. Of relevance to the racial focus of this study was the discovery that Black enrollees in Medicaid were more inclined to take advantage of screening for cervical cancer, breast cancer, colorectal cancer, and prostate cancer than were White enrollees. It was important to learn that primary care utilization as well as enrollees with a longer history of Medicaid enrollment were more commonly connected positively to cancer screening whereas co-occurring substance use disorder manifested a negative association with cancer screening. Continuous insurance coverage and ready access to primary care were suggested as positive ways of improving cancer screening rates among severe mental illness patients.

The extremely high rate of mortality among women with breast cancer is well and universally documented and with lung cancer and cardiovascular disease these three types of disease constitute the most abiding factors in mortality among women. What is not quite so thoroughly documented is the linkage between women with breast cancer who prior to that diagnosis were suffering from a preexisting mental illness and that linkage's relevance to the rate of mortality among these patients. A further factor of significance is that of breast cancer patients who are covered with Medicaid such that socioeconomic issues may constitute an integral component of this matrix of Medicaid insured women diagnosed with breast cancer with a preexisting mental illness. The complexity of this tripartite matrix constituted the impetus for the launching of a major databased study of this topic by Wayne R. Lawrence of the School of Public Health at the State University of New York. With eight colleagues from his own institution and medical professionals from the New York State Department of Health and the Albany Medical College, this team initiated a multi-level assessment of the convergence of these three factors, i.e., breast cancer, preexisting mental illness, and Medicaid recipients, in an attempt to identify the complexities of their linkage to mortality (Lawrence, Kuliszewski, Hosler, Leinung, et al., 2021). The intent was to determine to what extent a concerted effort should be put forth by the health care system in the treating of patients suffering with breast cancer with full cognizance of the relevance of the presence of mental illness in a Medicaid patient prior to the cancer diagnosis with an eye towards the reduction of the high rate of mortality among this category of patients.

During the period of time from 2004 to 2016 there were 10,444 women in the State of New York diagnosed with breast cancer over the age of 65 years on the claims records of Medicaid according to the New York State Registry. Based on a diagnosis record of at least three separate medical visits within a three year period prior to a breast cancer diagnosis, women were identified in this cohort who suffered from depression or a severe mental illness (SMI). The severe mental illnesses identified in this study included women suffering from schizophrenia, bipolar disorder, and unspecified psychiatric disorders. The team also gave a menopausal status estimate based on age 50 as the divide between pre- and post-menopausal status and calculated hazard ratios and confidence intervals based on Cox proportional hazards regression which was adjust to allow for confounders.

Not surprisingly but statistically validated was the discovery that preexisting serious mental illness patients experienced an all-cause and cancer-specific mortality rate far above patients with no SMI but no linkage between preexisting depression and mortality was verified. Also, among non-Hispanic White women a hazard ratio of 1.47 compared to non-Hispanic Asian/Pacific Islander women recorded a hazard ratio of 2.59 but the highest mortality hazard ratio existed for women with a preexisting serious mental disorder who were postmenopausal, obsess, and documented tobacco users. The findings were conclusion in determining that women who had a diagnostic history of a preexisting serious mental illness are clearly more susceptible to an elevated mortality hazard rate which led the researchers to suggest a closer monitoring of this classification of patient and they called for a coordinated cross-functional clinical involvement.

A conundrum is not uncommon in medical research and the fact that oncology records show that cancer patients with identified mental illness have a lower rate of survival than cancer patients without mental disorders constitutes one of the more baffling realities. The range of topics in oncology research is impressive but the study of the relationship between cancer and mental illness is one of those topics of research interest which commonly receives less attention. The need for a more refined databased study of this relationship is obvious and Ruth Cunningham and several of her colleagues at the Department of Public Health of the University of Otago in Wellington, New Zealand, set about to fill this void in information (Cunningham, Sarfati, et al., 2015). Concentrating its research interests specifically in New Zealand, this team focused upon breast and colorectal cancer registrations dating from 2006 to 2010. They chose to link their data to the psychiatric hospitalization records for adults in New Zealand during this time period for ages 18 to 64 years old.

The team used the Cox regression data in their assessment of the cancer-specific survival rates compared to the recent psychiatric service users and nonusers alike. Dividing the data participants into Group A (schizophrenia or bipolar affective disorder) and Group B (those choosing to use other mental health services), the researchers assessed the contributions of deprivation, comorbidity, and cancer stage at diagnosis as relevant variables. The database was substantial in that 8,762 patients had breast cancer and 4,022 had colorectal cancer. Of this group, 440 with breast cancer and 190 with colorectal cancer had been the recent recipients of psychiatric services. Following research protocol adjustments, they found that the risk of death from breast cancer had actually increased for Group A with a Hazard Ratio (HR) of 2.55 and from Group B with a Hazard Ratio of 1.62. Group A's HR for colorectal cancer registered 2.92 with later stage diagnoses contributing to the survival rates specifically. Comorbidity was found to be mutually impactful in both Group A and Group B.

The final and insightful conclusions from this massive databased study included the documentation for the high burden of physical disease linked to a delayed cancer diagnosis among psychotic disorder patients. The significantly worse cancer survival rate in New Zealand among psychiatric service users was both strikingly disturbing and contributed to a clarion call for national attention within the cancer treatment community and facilities.

The range of cancer research opportunities is seemingly endless such that specializations in sub-sets of available databases are continuing to emerge with the advancement of oncology research across the globe. From a research perspective, the range of research topics provides an arena within which virtually any serious constellation of medical variables may be analyzed with identification, diagnostic, and treatment protocols as the goal. Gender and age classification constitutes one of the most common fields of research. Xu Ji of the Department of Pediatrics at the Emory University School of Medicine in Atlanta, GA, has been joined by colleagues from several specialized institutions in Georgia to make a systematic enquiry into mental health issues characterizing non-elderly adult cancer patients and survival rates on a national level in the U.S. Xu Ji was joined by several colleagues from the Aflac Cancer and Blood Disorders Center at the Children's Healthcare of Atlanta, the Department of Health Policy and

Management at Emory University's Rollins School of Public Health, the Surveillance and Health Services Research division of the American Cancer Society, and the Department of Epidemiology at the Emory University Rollins School of Public Health in Atlanta, GA. (Xu Ji, Cummings, Marchak, Han, Mertens, 2020).

What Xu Ji and colleagues were cognizant of was the fact that age stratification of mental health issues could prove of great value in the assessing of adult cancer survival rates and that a national study of the U.S. would be possible owing to access to national data available from reliable databanks developed by the National Survey on Drug Use and Health. They chose to focus on the years 2015 to 2017 and they delineated the stratified categories based on ages covering three groupings of 18-34, 35-49, and 50-64 years of age. The outcome of an assessment of the mental health of these age groups specifically indicated the survival rate of adult cancer patients in each grouping. In making the analytical adjustments for the controlling of demographics and socioeconomic status with each grouping, these researchers compared the mental health outcomes between those participants in this study with a cancer history and those without a cancer history. Covering all three age groupings, the team studied the outcomes of the respondents covering the immediate past year involving any major depressive episodes, any reported serious psychological distress, instances of suicidal thoughts, plans and attempts, and any other identified mental illness or serious mental illness on record. These categories of outcome proved most helpful in the comparative analysis of the three groupings of respondents.

The database on which this team's study relied consisted of 112,952 respondents without a reported cancer and 2,656 cancer survivors within each of the 3 age groupings.

They found that the survivors across the age spectrum experienced an elevated prevalence of mental health issues in 5 of the 7 measurement categories listed above. Furthermore, the data showed that among the first age grouping (18-34), cancer survivors were more likely to experience major depressive episodes than non-cancer respondents (18.1% vs 9.6%), serious psychological distress (34.2% vs 17.9%) suicidal thoughts (10.5% vs 7.0%), other mental illnesses (41.1% vs 23.3%) and a serious mental illness (13.2% vs 5.9%) during the previous year. Though manifesting a smaller magnitude of variance, the team did find that similar survivor rates were found among the other two groupings but with less variance in magnitude. Young adult survivors (18-34) did report an elevated likelihood of mental health issues across all seven categories of outcome.

As anticipated, this massive databased study showed conclusively that there exists an elevated prevalence of mental health issues present among adult cancer survivors above the general population such that these findings have called attention to the need for a further intensified development of care strategies involving particularly early detection of mental illness among these three age groups and the need to cultivate a more vigorous treatment protocol for cancer survivors.

Tracking the cancer time-line from diagnosis to mortality has always been a monitoring agenda of oncologists and the concern to identify factors affecting the trajectory of a cancer is an enduring topic of research interest. The type of cancer from which a patient is suffering greatly informs the time-line for on-going treatment and comorbidity is always within the spectrum of interest and treatment. One of the leading types of comorbid complications in assessment and treatment of cancer is that of pre-existing mental health issues such as Severe Mental Illness (SMI) and psychiatric disorders.

To identify and examine barriers to cancer trajectories of patients constituted the research agenda of Terese Myhre Bentson of the Central Denmark Region of Aarhus, Denmark. This initiative resulted in the creation of a substantial team of oncologists and medical professionals from a range of medical institutions throughout Denmark with the specific purpose of seeking clarification to questions surrounding the nature and function of barriers in dealing with cancer trajectories for patients suffering from a pre-existing severe mental illness (Bentson, Floe, Bruun, Eriksen, et al., 2023).

This team of researchers began by performing a systematic review following the guidelines prescribed by PRISMA (PROSPERO ID). The aim was to specifically examining barriers at the three levels of patient/provider/system related to cancer trajectories of patients suffering from a pre-existing severe mental disorder concurrently to the cancer diagnosis. Because patients with a pre-existing severe mental illness are much less willing to accept guideline-recommended cancer treatment, documented studies show that these patients therefore have a much reduced rate of cancer survival compared to cancer patients who are not suffering from mental illness. These facts being well established, the team selected nine eligible studies from the PRISMA which conformed to the research agenda's specifications. They sought to identify and classify barriers to patients suffering from a mental disorder receiving treatment divided into three categories, viz., at the patient-level which included lack of self-care as well as the ability to recognize physical health issues; to provider-level barriers including the stigma of having a mental illness on the part of the health care professionals servicing the patient; and at the system-level barriers such a fragmented health care and the inevitable fallout from poor care.

Significant disparities in cancer care for patients with a mental disorder were identified in barriers at the levels of patient, provider, and system care impacting cancer trajectories for patients suffering from a mental illness. The team called for more research dealing specifically with the recognition of these barriers and the need to improve cancer trajectories for this particular category of cancer patient.

An abiding concern within the oncology research community is to what extent, if any, there is a relationship between the initial diagnosis of cancer and the appearance of a mental disorder not previously detected in the patient. A plethora of questions have emerged from this general observation and concern including a specific question regarding whether or not there is a measurable acceleration of tumor growth in a diagnosed patients presenting symptoms of mental illness and, if so, to what extent there might be a clear connection and linkage between a diagnosis of a cancer and the rapid growth of the tumor when linked to a mental disorders and the overall relevance of a concern for cancer-specific mortality. J. Zhu of the Medical Epidemiology Department of Karolinsk Institutet in Stockholm has raised these questions and has been joined by interested research colleagues from the school of medical sciences at Orebro University in Sweden, Harard T. H. Chan School of Public Health in Boston, the Health and Society Institute of the University of Oslo in Norway and the faculty of medicine at the University of Iceland (Zhu, Fang, Sjolander, Fall, Adami, and Valdimarsdottir, 2017). The specific focus of this research team was upon the first-onset of mental disorders following a cancer diagnosis and the resulting cancer-specific mortality. They focused their attention upon data provided by the Swedish Patient Register.

Focusing on a government-sponsored data base of cancer patients diagnosed between 2004 and 2009 (following through 2010), the team examined records for 244,262 cancer patients identified through the Swedish Patient Register from which all mental disorders which had been formally diagnosed were found. These records focused on mood disorders, anxiety disorders, and substance abuse disorders which commonly appear in the diagnosis of cancer patients. The team designed a classification system which allowed for a study of mental disorders divided into first-onset and recurrent mental disorders. The interest was in identifying the linkage between mental disorders after cancer diagnosis and cancer-specific mortality which included adjusting for age, sex, calendar period, educational level, cancer stage, and cancer type at diagnosis. The Cox regression was used to estimate multivariable hazard rations (HRs) with confidence intervals measured.

This research team was able to identify 11,457 patients following a cancer diagnosis who also presented symptoms of mood disorders, anxiety disorders, and substance abuse disorders with just over half of that number (n=7,236) were first-onset mental disorders. These first-onset mentally ill cancer patients were characterized at an elevated risk of cancer-specific mortality as compared to patients with a recurrent mental illness who experienced a much reduced mortality risk. Localized cancer patients rather than the more advanced cancer patients were much more susceptible to a cancer-specific mortality if experiencing a first-set mental illness. The overall findings led the team to call attention to the fact that cancer patients with first-onset common mental illness such as mood, anxiety, and substance abuse disorders were at an elevated risk of cancer-specific deaths and merited close monitoring by the health care team.

The complexity of the linkage between cancer and mental illness is recognized throughout the oncology world of diagnosis and treatment but beyond the documented reality that poor physical health is associated with severe mental illness, there is much uncertainty and confusion. The further area of concern is that of the relationship between mortality and cancer patients suffering from a mental disorder such that a composite study of the tripartite relationship of cancer, mental illness, and mortality constitutes a baffling yet intriguing area of specialized research. In order to bring clarity to this matrix of variables, Naomi Launders and her colleagues from the Division of Psychiatry at the University College London have ventured into these troubled waters with the intent of employing a massive database of information in order to investigate the linkage between severe mental illness with cancer and mortality in order to determine the relationship of premature mortality on cancer rates within the United Kingdom (Launders, Scolamiero, Osborn, Hayes, 2022). This particular approach to this complex issue was precipitated by the team's realization that to-date the findings have been inconclusively vague and documentation is sketchy and insufficient to make a sound assessment and judgment.

The team established a starting point for this research by using competing risk regression approaches to adjust for mortality from other causes than cancer. They commenced their analysis using primary care records for this UK-wide matched cohort study where they calculated both incidence and mortality rates among all cancers (bowel, lung, breast, prostate) in all patients with a documented severe mental illness and then compared that with cancer patients without a mental disorder.

Concentrating their databased study on 69,632 cancer patients with a diagnosed Severe Mental Illness (SMI), they found that the rate of all-cancer diagnoses diminished in patients registering also with a severe mental illness compared to patients without an SMI especially as regards patients with Schizophrenia. They further found that in taking account of premature mortality risks, the incidence remained lower but only in patients with schizophrenia. Also, they found that among all-cause mortality patients there was an elevated risk among SMI patients and cancer-specific mortality actually rose in patients with schizophrenia.

From this landmark databased study, the team was able to demonstrate that patients suffering from schizophrenia actually have a reduced rate of cancer diagnosis compared to an elevated all-cause and cancer-specific mortality rate following the diagnosis compared to patients without a severe mental illness. The troubling nature of their findings centered around the unexplained discovery that premature mortality does not fundamentally account for these differences such that barriers in cancer diagnosis and treatment relative to SMI and mortality must continue to be sought out through further databased studies. The significance of this study is a validation of this concern and justification for a clarion call for more research.

An inquiry into the relationship of cancer mortality and mental illness has been an abiding agenda from early in the history of modern oncology. That there has not been any reliable databased research validating or verifying a "causal" relationship between cancer and mental illness, the challenge has been to researchers to move away from a look at the medical and biochemical possibilities of a link between cancer and psychiatric disorders to a more refined and sophisticated assessment of the psychosocial spectrum of cancer. Since it has been more than once verified that cancer does not cause mental illness nor mental illness the cause of cancer, the search for the nature of the relationship between cancer mortality and mental disorders nevertheless constitutes an abiding point of research and controversy. To this end, Federico Chierzi of the Local Health Trust of Bologna, Italy, has put together a research team of medical oncologists and psychiatrists from the Local Health Trust of Bologna as well as from the Universities of Bologna and Ferrara for the purpose of exploring and explicating the nature of the relationship having discounted a bio-chemical causality. The research team began with the suggestion that patients suffering from what they chose to label "Common Mental Disorders (CMDs)" are more likely susceptible to a higher cancer mortality than the general public. Their interest focused upon the cancer-related mortality among patients with CMDs in an attempt to verify the types of cancer which are most predominant in this matrix.

Concentrating their databased study on the Emilia-Romagna region of Northern Italy, the researchers used the Regional Mental Health Registry to identify cancer patients who were 18 years old or older who had been diagnosed on the basis of an ICD9-CM for common mental disorders including particularly depressive and neurotic disorders) during a ten years period from 2008-2017. Mortality records were provided by the Regional Cause of Death Registry and these numbers were compared to the same regional population who did not have a Common Mental Disorder (CMD) diagnosis. The cancer mortality rates were drawn from 101,487 patients who were at the time suffering from CMDs (55.7% depression; 44.3% neurotic disorders) and 3,087 (37.8%) died from neoplasms. Given the fact that the established standard mortality ratio (SMR) was set at 1.82 while the SMR for all neoplasms was set at 2.08, patients of both genders suffering from both depressive and neurotic disorders actually registered an elevated risk of death from most cancer as compare to the regional population.

Therefore, the research team concluded, based on these numbers, that patients with CMDs actually do register a significantly elevated cancer mortality risk as compared to the general population. In this analysis they found that an elevated rate of mortality was demonstrated in a full spectrum of cancers linked to a wide assortment of etiologies. Finally and based on these findings, the team was insistent that the promotion of cancer awareness, prevention and treatment for patients suffering from psychiatric disorders be addressed robustly by the oncology and medical communities of all health care services within the region.

CHAPTER FOUR

Topical Issues linking Cancer and Mental Illness

Cancer and Tobacco; Pharmacology; Cancer Screening; Demoralization and Suicidality; Adolescent and Young Adult Cancer; Person-Centered Ca ncer Care

One of the characteristics of patients with a serious mental illness is the presence of other physically harmful activities and habits, even addictions such as liquor and tobacco, and because over half of all documented patients with a serious mental illness smoke, there is a direct correlation with the premature cancer deaths among this group of patients. The question as to what extent there might be some benefit in cancer patients suffering from a psychiatric disorder undergoing a cessation intervention program directed at tobacco smoking constituted a particular point of interest to Eleanor B. Staffens of the Department of Psychological Sciences at the University of Missouri in St. Louis, MO. In order to test the effectiveness of tobacco cessation interventionist programs among cancer patients during treatment, Staffens mobilized a team of distinguished medical professionals from the Memorial Sloan Kettering Cancer Center in New York with colleagues from the Massachusetts General Hospital and Harvard Medical School to address this question (Steffens, Park, Muzikaansky, Streck, et al., 2023). In light of the fact that over half of patients suffering from a serious mental illness are smokers which contributes to premature cancer deaths, Steffens and team believed that a cancer diagnosis might present a significant opportunity for clinical staff to assist the patient in the cessation of smoking. But, alas, most oncology trials have a tendency to exclude cancer patients with a diagnosed psychiatric disorder. So in order to fill this void in the research, this team chose to examine differences in engagement and tobacco cessation in a programed interventionist clinical trial.

In order to move ahead with this databased proposed study, the Steffens team called on two National Cancer Institute-designated Comprehensive Cancer Centers to recruit some 303 cancer patients who were smokers of which 10% were suffering from a serious mental illness such as a major depressive disorder, bipolar disorder, and schizophrenia spectrum disorders. Relying upon a comparison of behaviors based on self-reporting smoking habits, the team also documented patient attitudes and beliefs relative to the issue of the cessation of smoking as well as rates of attempted completion, engagement, and smoking abstinence focusing on the diagnosed patients with cancer both with and without a serious mental illness. After a six month hiatus following the trial period, the team engaged in qualitative interviews based on the barriers and facilitators to tobacco cessation among a random sample of patients who were diagnosed with a serious mental illness.

The team found that there was no measurable difference between participating patients with a serious mental illness who were motivated to quit smoking as those participating patients who did not suffer from a mental illness. Furthermore, they found that patients with an SMI were more or less equally able to participate in a tobacco treatment trial and thus benefit from tobacco treatment care as those patients who had no SMI.

These clinical findings did suggest, however, that cancer patients suffering from a serious mental illness were actually able to fully engage in as well as benefit from the tobacco cessation trial integrated into their cancer treatment care. They found that the cancer diagnosis actually provided an occasion to assist the patient suffering from a serious mental illness with smoking cessation referrals and treatment protocols. The Steffens research group came to the conclusion that pragmatic supportive oncology trials which also included a diversified patient population with a serious mental illness can prove helpful and informative in educating the care delivery medical personnel when dealing with cancer smoking patients with an SMI.

A team of medical professionals at the University of Ferrara's Institute of Psychiatry in Italy under the leadership of the internationally acclaimed research oncologist Luigi Grassi (Grassi, et al., 2014) was early in calling attention to the need for further and more comprehensive data-based research on the efficacy of pharmacological treatment of cancer patients suffering from identified psychiatric disorders focusing upon pharmacotherapy as a relative new and advancing field of treatment. These researchers recognized that upwards of 30% of cancer patients, particularly those in advanced stages, qualify for psychiatric diagnoses of such disorders as depression, anxiety, stress-related syndromes, adjustment disorders, sleep disorders and delirium.

Generally recognized within the medical community of the efficacy of some carefully screened psychotropic medicals for the treatment of identified psychiatric disorders, recent developments in psychopharmacological research has shown the effectiveness of such drugs in the treatment of cancer-related symptoms such as pain, hot flashes, pruritus, nausea and vomiting, fatigue, and even some cognitive impairments. As a service to research professionals in psychiatric oncology, Grassi and colleagues did an extensive investigation of the major leading databased studies current at the time of their research including MEDLINE, Embase, PsycLIT, PsycINFO, and the Cochrane Library in an effort to provide a generalized summary of the efficacy of pharmacotherapies used in cancer-related psychiatric disorders.

A major feature in the integration of psychiatry and oncology has been the result of the accelerated development and use of psychotropic medications in the treatment of mental illness in the last 50 years owing to the closure of state-run psychiatric hospitals and the rise of a refined professionalization of psychotherapy. The emergence of psychiatric oncology has been the direct result of this integration and the cancer patient has consistently been the beneficiary of this development. However, and in light of the relative newness of the integration of psychiatric medication in the overall treatment of cancer patients, there has been a lag in the research focused on the long term effects of certain psychotropic medications in the treatment protocol and the long term effects of such on the cancer patient. Blanaid M. Hicks of the Centre for Public Health at the Royal Victoria Hospital in Belfast, N.I., has put together a team of likeminded medical professionals from the Belfast City Hospital and Queen's University of Belfast to create a databased study of the relationship of psychotropic medication and cancer mortality with special attention to the mortality of breast cancer patients. This focused specialization has until the time of this study been overlooked or systematically avoided owing to possible political as well as economic constraints and considerations (Hicks, Busby, Mills, O'Neil, et al., 2020).

The impetus for Hicks and company's interest in this topic centered around the realization that in spite of the fact that it is well known within the oncology community that the use of certain antipsychotic medications actually contribute to the elevation of prolactin in the patient, a hormone linked to the etiology of breast cancer, there is the startling absence of any serious databased study of the use of anti-psychologic medications in breast cancer patients. The absence of real quantitative data addressing this issue is disturbing owing to the fact that there might be a link between antipsychotic medication and an elevated risk of cancer-specific mortality among this particular class of cancer type. More was needed and Hicks and team set out to fill the void of information through a massive databased study. They began with a cohort database of 23,695 women recently diagnosed with breast cancer covering the dates from January 1, 1998 to December 31, 2012. This cohort database was provided by the United Kingdom Clinical Practice Research Datalink to the English cancer-registries. The team followed these cancer patients until September 30, 2015, using the Cox proportional hazards models to actually calculate the hazard ratios (HRs) and confidence intervals (Cis) of breast cancer mortality. They specifically sought to compare cancer patients using antipsychotic medical with cancer patients who did not use such psychotropic medication as well as patients involved in prolactin elevating medicaton. The danger, of course, was the possibility of confounding their findings such that their analyses were repeatedly limited to cancer patients with a documented history of severe mental illness.

The data analysis was restricted to an 848 patient cohort who were receiving an antipsychotic medication during the trial period such that 162 of these patients died of breast cancer. The restriction was for patients with documented and diagnosed severe mental illness in which the patients were recipients of an antipsychotic medication and subject to breast cancer mortality. As compared to patients not receiving antipsychotic drugs, those who did receive such medication experienced an elevated risk of breast cancer specific mortality. However and somewhat baffling was the fact that the mortality rate did not adhere to a dose response linkage. The team found that a confounding by indication was finally lacking in their study of this cohort of breast cancer patients owing to the fact that though the use of antipsychotic medication was linked with an elevation of breast cancer-specific mortality, they could not verify that there was any direct indication of a dose response related to patients suffering from severe mental illness. Finally, the team was led to point out that studies of confounding by indication are crucial in attempting to understand the linkage between medication and mortality in cancer patients keeping in mind the presence of an implicit bias involving the confounding by indication.

Less than a decade ago, Lara C. Weinstein of the Department of Family and Community Medicine at the Thomas Jefferson University in Philadelphia (Weinstein, et al., 2016) with several institutional colleagues from her own university as well as from the Columbia School of Social Work in New York reported an appalling scarcity of any serious databased studies addressing issues related to cancer screening, prevention, and treatment protocols of individuals also suffering with a mental illness. Referencing the existing bibliographic citations, limited as this field of research is, Weinstein points out that the past history of cancer in the United States saw an appalling disparity in the death rate of cancer patients with mental illness compared to the national average within the general population. And, as this research team emphasizes, this disparity is linked to actually preventable and treatable chronic conditions.

In view of the fact that cancer deaths constitute the second leading cause of death in the U.S. (second only to heart disease), this team investigated individual lifestyle factors such as smoking and limited treatment access for cancer patients with mental illness as relevant contextual and systems-level factors driving health disparities within this matrix of cancer patients. In the team's integrative review of the literature addressing the three major components of this investigation, i.e., cancer prevention, screening, and treatment for mentally ill patients, they were unable to verify any significantly effective treatment protocol which has been developed to address system-wide this problem. However, at the individual level some measurable help has been identified in dealing with comorbid issues such as tobacco addiction and obesity.

An embarrassingly troubled observation made by the research team was that of all of the literature in the field they reviewed, they were able to only actually identify one published article in the scholarly medical journals considering evidence-based intervention relative to the screening and treatment protocols of cancer patients with mental illness. Drawing from their own professional training and experience as well as a review summary of existing literature, they were insistent upon the accelerated need for more direct research at the individual, interpersonal, organization, community, and policy levels if any progress is to be realized in improving the overall assessment and treatment of cancer patients with mental illness.

In the assessment and diagnosis of a cancer, a particularly helpful component of this care of the patient is the knowledge of whether or not the patient was suffering from a pre-existing mental illness in advance of the cancer diagnosis

particularly linked to factors related to cancer-specific mortality. Gathering of this particular statistical package proved of great benefit in the overall assessment of the care and treatment of cancer patients with mental illness histories. Faculty members of the various Departments of Surgery, Surgical Oncology, Medical Oncology, Palliative Medicine, and Internal Medicine at The Ohio State University Wexner Medical Center were led by Anghela Z. Paredes in an orchestrated effort to formalize a more comprehensive understanding of the relationship of pre-existing mental illness with cancer mortality particularly, in this study, of pancreatic cancer (Paredes, Hyer, Tsilimigras, Palmer, et al., 2021). The driving concern for this team of researchers was the virtual absence of any significantly databased understanding of the linkage between pre-existing mental illness and long-term outcomes of cancer treatment. Since one in every 12 patients suffering from pancreatic cancer also was suffering from a pre-existing mental illness, the urgency of this study was self-evident and pancreatic cancer patients with a pre-existing mental illness necessarily faced the prospects of a diminished overall life expectancy as well as a declining quality of life.

Focusing their attention upon data provided by the SEER-Medicare database, the team examined individuals who had been diagnosed with pancreatic adenocarcinoma and these individuals were classified as suffering from a mental illness as identified by the ICD9/10CM code for anxiety, depression, bipolar disorder, schizophrenia and other unspecified psychotic disorders. The data base consisted of 54,234 Medicare beneficiaries who had been identified with pancreatic cancer of which 1 in 12 (n=4,793, 8.83%) had previously been diagnosed with a mental illness. Of this number, over 80% (n=4,029) were suffering from anxiety or depression while less than 20%

(n=764) were diagnosed with bipolar/schizophrenic disorders. Based on a multivariable analysis of patients who had been diagnosed with early stage cancer, a reported reduced Odds Rates (OR) to undergo cancer-directed surgery characterized 22% of the patients suffering from anxiety/depression and 46% suffering from bipolar/schizophrenic disorders. In addition to which these cancer patients diagnosed with a pre-existing history of bipolar/schizophrenic disorders reported a 20% higher rate of risk for all-cause mortality and 27% with a higher risk rate of pancreatic cancer-specific mortality as compared to patients without a mental illness history. The findings were clear that pancreatic cancer patients suffering from mental illness were more susceptible to an overall cancer-specific mortality rate than those without a mental illness.

Developments within cancer research have been coming fast over the past few decades but not all technological advancements were readily and quickly embraced. Cancer screening and early detection has its own checkered history of development and adoption within the medical community. As early as the 1920s, there was a movement to introduce screening for Pap test led by Geoge Papanicolaou who first applied this new procedure to cervical cancer. Though initially the medical community was reluctant to embrace this new approach (not an uncommon characteristics of the traditionalism in medical practice) following the American Cancer Society's endorsement of the test during the 1960s screening has become commonplace. The test, however, is even now not universally available or applied and not available to all cancer patients relative to their socioeconomic status, nationality, and particularly their mental health. Since the introduction of screening for cervical cancer, for example, the mortality rate has dropped 50%. Thanks to a distinguished team of oncologists at the Johns Hopkins School of Medicine in Baltimore under the leadership of Karly A. Murphy, a major database study was launched in 2021 to address the issues surrounding cancer screening for adults both with a serious mental illness and those without in order that a comparative analysis might be conducted (Murphy, Stone, Presskreischer, et al., 2021).

As has been being discussed in this overview of the relationship of cancer to mental illness, there is a universally validated documentation that cancer is the second leading cause of death in the world next only to heart disease. Cancer patients suffering from a serious mental illness are more likely to die 10 to 20 years earlier than the average person in the general population. In spite of the massive documentation addressing these realities, Murphy and colleagues at the Johns Hopkins School of Medicine were troubled by the general disregard for or fundamental absence of studies examining the nature of the relationship between cancer screening and serious mental illness in the general population, a research void crying out for investigation and resolution. Another related issue which was of interest to this research team was the commonly noted variance in attitudes of clinical oncologists regarding the perceptions of the role of cancer screening for patients suffering from mental illness.

A refined focused research was employed including a mixed methods approach using data provided by the MarketScan commercial insurance administrative claims data departments covering 2010 through 2017 including semi-structured clinician interviews. For purposes of this study the research team chose to circumscribe the definitional parameters of serious mental illness (SMI) to be restricted to schizophrenia and bipolar disorder. In this quantitative analysis, they used a multivariate logistic regression approach to calculate the likelihood that patients with cervical, breast, colorectal, or prostate cancer suffering from serious mental illness would actually receive screening. Using a hybrid deductive/inductive approach to transcript records, the team engaged in semi-structured interviews with primary care physicians and psychiatrists.

They found that comparative to cancer patients without a serious mental illness, patients with an SMI were actually less likely to have undergone screening for cervical cancer, breast cancer, colorectal cancer, or prostate cancer. This finding led the team to propose 5 factors which helps to understand this discrepancy leading to lower rates of cancer screening among patients suffering from serious mental illness, viz., access to care, available support, other issues taking priority over the care practice, failures in communication across the board with patients and medical personnel, and essential issues and concerns of the individual patient. Based on this extensive study, the research team was convinced that further enhancement of cancer screening among patients with serious mental illness will certainly call for a concerted effort on the part of all communities involved in cancer care if the current blocking patterns are to be removed.

As has been consistently shown throughout this investigation into the nature and scope of the relationship between cancer and mental illness, from a medical and health care perspective it is not enough to address the biomedical issues involved in oncology for the patient is clearly more than plasma and tissue. Since the work of the early psychiatric oncologists at the leading cancer centers of research in the U.S. and abroad, it has been self-evident that the psychosocial spectrum of cancer care must always be thought of and recognized as a major component of overall cancer assessment, diagnosis, and treatment. Sigrun Vehling at the Princess Margaret Cancer Centre of the University Health Network in Toronto, Canada, has put together a team of psychiatrists and medical psychologists for the purpose of explore the complexities of this linkage. It is evident in clinical studies of what is commonly called "demoralization" among patients suffering from cancer is linked that of mental disorders and particularly suicidal ideation. (Vehling, Kissane, Lo, et al., 2017). The team began with an agreed-upon circumscribed definition of the term demoralization as that of "a state of being in which the individual experiences a perceived inability to cope with life's demands manifesting an overall sense of disheartenment and a loss of hope and meaning in life." The challenge to the research team was to be able to devise a method of analysis which provided a means of differentiating between demoralization and that of independence from demoralization. In relationship to mental disorders and suicidal ideation, evaluating the fundamental characteristics of demoralization in defining distress within severe mental illness is difficult but crucial.

The team used a cross-sectional sample of 430 mixed cancer patients in an effort to compare the relative risk (RR) for mental disorders which are commonly associated with demoralization with self-reported depression on the part of the individual participants. The standard method for assessing demoralization is by means of the Demoralization Scale (DS). By using the standardized Composite International Diagnostic Interview-Oncology (CIDI-), they were able to check the 4-week prevalence of mood, anxiety, and adjustment disorders as well as suicidal ideation. Finally, they measured depressive symptoms using the Patient Health Wquestionnaire-9 (PHQ-9).

Of the 430 cancer patients being studies, they found that 21% of them registered a clinically relevant level of demoralization with some 7% measuring a demoralization co-occurrence of a mood/anxiety disorder. Furthermore, even in the absence of any measurable mood/anxiety disorder, the respondents showed 14% as demoralized with both demoralization and adjustment disorders appearing concurrently at 2% of the study group. For any measurable mood/anxiety disorders there was a 4.0 relative risk involved with patients suffering from demoralization and a 3.0 risk factor for those with depression. Excluding depression which was not present, demoralization was linked to a significantly elevated risk factor for suicidal ideation when controlling for any identifiable mental disorder. The team discovered that in light of the fact that clinical demoralization often occurs separate from any identifiable mental disorder in cancer patients and is not infrequently present in suicidal ideation, they determined that demoralization should be considered a meaningfully relevant concept in identifying psychological distress symptoms susceptible to psychiatric intervention.

Within the general context of investigating the nature of the relationship between cancer and mental illness, there are a range of variables which must be factored into any generalized observations. Granted the international consensus regarding the relationship of cancer and mental illness is that there is a psychosocial dynamic descriptive of this interplay. There is the recognition that there has not yet been any validation of a biochemical linkage between cancer and mental illness such that the psychiatric disorders manifested by cancer patients during the diagnostic and treatment period was either present in advance of the diagnosis or emerged as a result of the emotional stress produced by a cancer diagnosis. What further complicates these inquiries is the introduction of the cancer patient's experience of surgery while also displaying a mental illness. This tripartite configuration of cancer, mental illness, and surgery constituted the driving impetus for a research project initiated led by J. Madison Hyer at the Wesner Medical Center and Solove Research Institute of The Ohio State University. With a select group of surgeons and oncologists, Hyer launched a massive databased study of the relationship between mental illness and the cancer surgical patient relative to the elevation of suicidal ideation, a topic very little specifically investigated until this study was conducted in 2021 with a team of medical professionals from the Wesner Medical Center (Hyer, Kelly, Paredes, et al., 2021).

Research is replete with databased studies of the linkage between mental illness such as depression and the elevated risk of suicide and suicidal ideation. What the Hyer team set out to do in this database study was to identify the nature of the linkage between mental illness and suicidal ideation when manifested among surgical cancer patients, a specialized category of patients. Cancer and mental illness are themselves distressingly troubling but the added variable of cancer surgery elevates the distress level exponentially. The team chose to focus on Medicare beneficiaries who suffered from a resection of lung, esophageal, pancreatic, colon, and rectal cancer and to further refine this study they divided these patients in the study into three groups, i.e., no mental illness, anxiety and/or depression disorders, and bipolar/schizophrenic disorders. Research of this Medicare database of the 211,092 patient beneficiaries who actually received surgery for their cancer, 270 of these patients reported suicidal ideation with a registered antecedent mental illness diagnosis recording an elevated increase in suicidal ideation. Using a multivariable analysis, the studies showed that patients with anxiety only, depression only, anxiety and depression, and bipolar/schizophrenia all reported a measured elevation of suicidal ideation. Based on these findings and the statistical evidence that one in 370 Medicare beneficiaries suffering from cancer who experienced a surgical procedure manifested suicidal ideation such that clearly this study demonstrated that an antecedent mental illness diagnosis constituted an elevated risk for suicidal ideation.

The profoundly high level of connectivity between suicide and cancer has been documented extensively as in my recent book, *Cancer and Suicide: A Resource Compendium of Published Research, 1978-2023* (John H. Morgan, Wyndham Hall Press, N. Fort Myers, FL, 2023). Where there is still much work to be done in psychiatric oncology is the linkage between cancer and suicide among patients also suffering from mental illness. This present book, *Cancer and Mental Illness: A Decade of Published Research in Review* (N. Fort Myers, FL., 2024 forthcoming) has focused research specifically upon the relationship of cancer to mental illness. Sigrun Vehling from the Department of Medical Psychology at the University Medical Center in Hamburg along with colleagues in oncology from his own university and that of the University Medical Center of Leipzig have joined forces in examining more closely the relationship of death thoughts and suicidality found in cancer patients who have been diagnosed suffering from mental disorders (Vehling, Mehnert-Theuerkauf, Glaesmer, et al., 2021). Recognizing the linkage between a cancer diagnosis and a measurable elevation in the increased risk of suicide, this team examined such subcategories of suicidal behavior as thoughts of death, death wishes, and suicidal ideation as these behavioral matrices were linked with patients suffering from mental disorders as well as demographic and disease-related characteristics.

Using the standardized Composite International Diagnostic Interview-Oncology (CIDI-O), they undertook to analyze 2,141 cancer patients consisting of an assessment of a documented 4-weeks-prevalence of thoughts of death, wish to die, suicidal ideation, suicide plans, and lifetime suicide attempts as recorded in the database. They went further and recorded the 4-weeks-prevalences of mood, anxiety, adjustment, somatoform, substance use, and disorders linked to general medical conditions of the subjects being studied including latent class analyses (LCA). This instrument assisted the team in identifying three classes of cancer patients with some level of suicidality. Class I (89% of 2,141 patients) demonstrated no suicidality while Class II (being just under 7% of the test group) displayed thoughts of death without suicidal ideation. Class III (4.1% of the test group) did manifest thoughts of death, suicidal ideation, and suicidal plans with actual death wishes appearing in both Class II and Class III. These two classes (II and III) displayed a substantially higher rate of risk for all types of mental disorder, adjustment disorder, and mood disorder compared to Class I. The team found that cancer patients who suffered from mental disorders were equally distributed in Class I and Class II but patients with an incurable cancer diagnosis were substantially more likely in Class II and less so in Class III.

In conclusion to their study, the team of researchers was insistent that cancer patients who have displayed suicidal ideations are not specifically described as having a mental disorder and, therefore, further study is clearly needed in order to understand to what extent there might be an identifiable link between a cancer diagnosis and suicidal ideation on the part of patients suffering from a mental illness.

Mortality and cancer are always part of any serious clinical study in oncology and the factors leading to death during a patient's experience with cancer constitute a fundamental topic of research and discussion. Because cancer is a leading cause of death in the world and commonly related to a comorbidity, oncologists are eager to assess the dynamics of the interaction between cancer and other health factors including the psychosocial spectrum of cancer. The emergence of psychiatric oncology is a direct result of this growing awareness of the complex relationship between a patient with cancer from the point of diagnosis onwards and the patient's emotional well-being necessarily constitutes a significant field of research. Combine the factors of cancer and psychiatric assessment with that of suicidal ideation and the patient and the medical care team are presented with a fascinating and complex array of comorbid phenomena. However and even in light of the universal recognition of the central importance of understanding a cancer patient's experience of a mental disorder in the midst of dealing with a cancer diagnosis, there is little databased research on the relationship of a cancer patient with a psychiatric disorder or mental illness and the ever-present reality of suicidality issues. A comprehensive study of cancer and suicide was my 2023 book *Cancer and Suicide: A Resource Compendium of Published Research (1978-2023)* but mental illness was not dealt with in that book in anticipation of this current work.

In order to more explicitly explicate and delineate the complex convergence of contributing factors to a resulting suicide in the life of a cancer patient suffering from a mental disorder, Geoffrey D. Kahn of the Center for Health Policy &

Health Services Research at the Henry Ford Health hospital in Detroit, MI, has put together a distinguished team of oncologists and psychiatric professionals from a wide range of American medical institutions for the specific purpose of dealing with this challenging topic (Kahn, Tam, Felton, Westphal, et al., 2023). This team focused on the reality that cancer patients are recognized as particularly susceptible to a risk of suicide but the real issue is the need for a deeper understanding of the linkage and interaction between cancer patients and a psychiatric diagnosis leading up to the act of suicide. One notion which the team explored was that there is a synergistic relationship between cancer and a psychiatric diagnosis and to finally dislodge this notion based on a databased study would go a long way in advancing a clearer understanding of that relationship devoid of a synergistic linkage.

This research team created a retrospective case-control study based on aggregated data gathered from the electronic medical records from nine different healthcare systems participating in the Mental Health Research in Michigan. They used the ICD-9 codes for the purposes of identifying patients diagnosed one year in advance of their suicide (N=3,330) or matching index dated for controls (N=297,034). Based on a conditional logistic regression model, the researchers used this model to identify and evaluate the differences in cancer patients and psychiatric diagnoses using cases and controls for comparison including sex and age. Excluding cancer patients without a concurrent psychiatric disorder, cancer patients with a lower average of 5-year survival rates were linked to a significantly high relative risk but patients with cancer with a survival rate of 70% or over actually conferred no increased risk of suicide. However, cancer patients with a psychiatric disorder diagnosis were at an elevated risk of suicide but there was actually no added risk to the patient for suicide when a concurrent cancer diagnosis occurred.

What was somewhat liberating to this team researching the tripartite composite of cancer, mental illness, and suicide was the databased verification that no evidence could be found that there actually exists a synergistic relationship between cancer itself and a psychiatric diagnosis. Rather, they found that cancer patients suffering from a concurrent psychiatric disorder stayed at the highest risk level for suicide irrespective of the cancer disease location in the body based on a strong free link between psychiatric diagnoses and suicide. Finally, the researchers were able to verify their pursuit of an explanation for why there exists an elevated suicide risk among cancer patients with a worse prognosis but not suffering concurrently from a psychiatric illness.

Psychiatric oncology as the professional perspective on the psychosocial spectrum of cancer care has distinguished itself over the past 50 years by drawing attention, not away from the biomedical character of cancer but to an inclusive approach to the cancer patient which includes all aspects of patient care from the clinical biomedical side of cancer to the psychosocial character of the overall patient's life. A considerably important feature of psychiatric oncology is demonstrated in its effective differentiation between the various age groups of cancer patients, from infancy and childhood to geriatric patients. Within this spectrum, there are subsets and one of the most researched subset is that of adolescent and young adult patients (AYA). A major initiative at the Sloan-Kettering Cancer Institute in New York undertaken by Dr. Jimmy Holland in the 1970s has led to an international movement focusing upon the psychosocial spectrum of cancer care designed specifically as a compliment and aid to medical oncology. This movement, embodied in the distinguished international publication, *Psychooncology*, has provided a platform for international sharing of specialized research in this area illustrated by a team of oncologists at several major German universities. Kristina Geue of the University Medical Center in Leipzig, Germany, has been joined by a team of distinguished oncologists throughout Germany with the intent of focusing upon the prevalence of mental disorders and their resulting psychosocial distress manifestations among German adolescent and young adult cancer patients (Geue, Brahler, Faller, Harter, et al., 2018).

A nationally accessed database of 302 AYA cancer patients (167 completed the CIDI-O) provided the research team with the opportunity of studying the prevalence of mental disorders within the test group covering a three leveled spans of time, i.e., 4-weeks, 1 year, and lifetime who were suffering from diagnosed psychological distress factors identified within these Adolescent and Young Adult (AYA) cancer study. Working with a database of over four million cancer patients who had volunteered to participate in an epidemiological study covering a range of major tumor types, the research team included in their study an AYA subsample of 15- to 39-year olds who had been diagnosed within the previous five years. Using a depression screener (PHQ-9), all participants were assessed and subsequently 50% of those participants scoring below the pre-set cutoff point of 9 as well as all other participants scoring above 9 were evaluated with the instrument Composite International Diagnostic Interview for Oncology (CIDI-O) as well as all patients completing the GAD-7 for anxiety screening.

Of the total AYA test group involved in this study of psychological distress, almost 30% had an increase in depression symptoms measured by the PHQ-9 with 20% actually experiencing an increase in their anxiety symptoms as indicated by the GAD-7. In tracking the levels of psychological distress among the study patients, the team found that in considering both gender and age of the participants it showed that women and the older adolescent and young adults manifested a higher level of distress with the four-week prevalence of mental illnesses registering nearly 50% while anxiety manifested nearly 25% and adjustment disorders just under 14%. What was encouraging from a social concerns perspective was the discovery that alcohol dependence registered the lowest prevalence rate at below 1% of the study group with somatoform disorders showing 3.7%. Covering the full range of time considerations the one-year prevalence registered at 55.4% and the lifetime prevalence at 69.5%. It was the intent of this study to emphasize the value of sensitizing practitioners and clinicians to the presence of mental disorders within the AYA population generally and to call attention to the need for psychosocial interventions within oncological practice in order to further enrich the mental health care and treatment of AYA cancer patients at all level of medical care and attention.

An interesting area of research in the past few years has been that of the etiology of mental illness in cancer patients within the scope of the question as to whether or not and/or to what extent a cancer diagnosis itself might have precipitated a psychological stress point such that a mental illness emerges or is produced. This point of inquiry constitutes a major area of concern for the oncology professionals who often encounter an upsurge of stress and anxiety at the time of a cancer diagnosis which potentially could account for a rise in a level of emotional distress classified as a mental disorder. Documentation regarding cancer diagnosis and the utilization of mental health services has commonly been taken from studies of primary care rather than actual healthcare related data based on medical claims. To address this nuanced distinction. Sandra Salm of the Faculty of Medicine at the University of Cologne was joined by several of her colleagues to make a formalized inquiry into the relevance and/or significance of this distinction (Salm, Blaschke, Ihle, Schubert, et al., 2021). The relevance of this study had the potential of making a significant impact upon the agencies involved in providing health care to cancer patients based on whether they utilized claims services or primary care services as the initial point of seeking help.

This research team launched their investigation by examining statutory health insurance claims from 2011 to 2014 which included cancer patients with a mental disorder who had taken advantage of the mental health services calculated in a time frame for the first quarter of the study time and three subsequent quarters of that same time frame. They then assessed the predictive value of such variables as sex, age group, and tumor of cancer patients with a mental disorder based on a clinical diagnosis. Within the framework of the 12-month prevalence of a mental disorder among cancer patients, just over 30% manifested depression, just over 10% showed anxiety disorders, and just under 10% displayed post-traumatic stress/adjustment disorder. Of this group of patients, 65.9% took advantage of outpatient psychotherapy with 43% utilizing psychopharmacological drug prescriptions at least once. The male patient demonstrated a substantially lower chance of a mental disorder diagnosis following a cancer diagnosis and this study found that a higher rate of depression and a lower rate of

PTSD/AD characterized patients with a prevalence of a mental disorder.

Not just disparity but timing consistently proves of significant relevance in the care and treatment of cancer. We have examined a number of studies in which disparity of treatment is linked to the presence of a serious mental illness or psychiatric disorder in a patient such that the survival rate of the patient is directly impacted by the linked relationship of diagnosis and mental health of the patient. However, not inconsequential as a contributing factor in the survival and mortality of the cancer patient is its link to the actual timing of the diagnosis and the commencing of treatment. As in the case with many if not most health situations, the timing of the medical response to a presenting illness can and often does prove profoundly consequential to the patient's survival prospects. Pedro Cespedes of the Department of Nursing in the Faculty of Nursing and Chiropody at the Spanish University of Valencia has put together a team of colleagues to specifically address the issues of survival linked to the factor of delay in the diagnostic assessment of breast and colorectal cancer patients who were suffering from a severe mental disorder (Cespedes, Sanchez-Martinez, Lera-Calatayud, et al., 2020).

Published databased research has consistently demonstrated that cancer patients with severe mental illness are much more likely to experience a poor cancer prognosis which leads to a higher rate of mortality than the general public. Cespedes and colleagues chose to investigate whether or not and/or to what extent a delay in early detection constituted a measurable factor in a lessening of survival rates. They point out in this study that in Spain, the country of research focus, there is an extensive screening program for both breast and colorectal cancer but what is absent is any data focusing on the relevance of early diagnostic detection for individuals suffering from severe mental disorders. This void in databased studies they chose to address.

The research team's approach was clear and simple, namely, to compare data reflecting the severity of breast and colorectal cancers at the time of diagnosis found in individuals with severe mental illness with those who manifested no signs of any mental disorder. Drawing data for analysis from an electronic medical records repository for Eastern Spain, the study was based on an observational, retrospective, case-control investigation. In this database, there were a total of 111 cancer patients of which 75 suffered from breast cancer and 36 from colorectal cancer. Patients with mental disorders were significantly higher in relative risk at the time of diagnoses if showing an advanced tumor stage of development for both breast cancer and colorectal cancer. The pivotal factor was linked to an advanced stage of cancer development at the time of diagnosis for patients with a previous mental disorder and of an older age. Consistently, their data showed that patients at an advanced stage of cancer development with severe mental illness manifested an elevated risk of being diagnosed with either breast cancer or colorectal cancer. In their final comment, the research team called for an orchestrated acceleration in the quality of cancer screening for early detection and treatment for cancer patients suffering from severe mental disorders owing to the present poor state of the institutional response to this group of patients. They believed that a coalition of mental health professionals, screening and oncology nurses could be of real service in the improvement of quality care for these patients from screening to treatment.

CONCLUDING REMARKS

The complexities of cancer research and treatment are legion and constitute a massive confluence of specializations within the medical profession as well as medical institutions. The complexities of mental illness likewise constitute a profoundly variegated confluence of psycho-behavioral as well as biomedical factors such that attempts to treat mental illness in the absence of medicine have constituted an on-going challenge to both medicine and psychiatry. To attempt a convergence of medicine and psychiatry is an endeavor worthy of both admiration and caution. That cancer and mental illness are linked is not a recent discovery and the preceding exercise in assessing and evaluating over 125 scholarly papers in the medical journals stands as a witness to this challenge. That we have shown the linkage between cancer and mental illness is indisputable and the profoundly expansive illustration of the extreme lengths to which the medical research community has gone stands as a testimony to the honor and value of databased and collaborative research in the interest of truth and practical application of scientific findings.

It is hoped that what has been done in this monograph wherein a host of leading scholarly papers have been surveyed and explicated showing the range and depth of medical research based on data analysis is demonstration of the merits of research and the insightful findings shown in these papers. Research conducted throughout the world in major medical institutions led by internationally distinguished medical practitioners and researchers is reflective of the quality of care in assessing and evaluating the practice of cancer care for patients suffering from mental illness. The task is great and the challenge has been well met by leaders in the field of psychiatric oncology wherein the psychosocial spectrum of cancer care is embodied in the overall holistic approach to medical practice. Both oncologists and behavioral scientists have demonstrated the efficacy of such collaboration and this monograph is illustrative of the value of such cooperation within the professions of oncology and psychiatry.

APPENDICES

A. GLOSSARY OF TERMS AND DATABASED STUDIES UTILIZED IN THIS STUDY*

Acceptance and Commitment Therapy (ACT)

Acceptance and commitment therapy is a form of psychotherapy, as well as a branch of clinical behavior analysis. It is an empirically based psychological intervention that uses acceptance and mindfulness strategies along with commitment and behavior-change strategies to increase psychological flexibility.

Adjuvant Therapy (AT)

This treatment targets cancer cells that primary cancer treatment did not destroy. Having adjuvant therapy means more time spent in cancer treatment, but reduces the chances of having the same cancer again. Adjuvant therapy is often used as follow-up treatment for breast, colon and lung cancers.

Adolescent and Young Adult (AYA)

Adolescent and young adult oncology is a branch of medicine that deals with the prevention, diagnosis, and treatment of cancer in adolescent and young adult (AYA) patients aged 16–40.

Adenocarcinoma

This is a type of cancer that starts in mucus-producing (glandular) cells. Many organs have these types of cells and adenocarcinoma can develop in any of these organs.

AJCC stage I-IV breast cancer

Stage 0 is a pre-cancerous or marker condition, either ductal carcinoma in situ (DCIS) or lobular carcinoma in situ (LCIS). Stages 1–3 are within the breast or regional lymph nodes. Stage 4 is 'metastatic' cancer that has a less favorable prognosis since it has spread beyond the breast and regional lymph nodes.

Angiogenesis

The formation of new blood vessels. This process involves the migration, growth, and differentiation of endothelial cells, which line the inside wall of blood vessels. The process of angiogenesis is controlled by chemical signals in the body.

Annual Cost per Patient Linear Model (ACPLM)

The term linear model is used in different ways according to the context. The most common occurrence is in connection with regression models and the term is often taken as synonymous with linear regression model.

Antipsychotics

Previously known as neuroleptics and major tranquilizers, antipsychotics are a class of psychotropic medication primarily used to manage psychosis (including delusions, hallucinations, paranoia or disordered thought), principally in schizophrenia but also in a range of other psychotic disorders. They are also the mainstay, together with mood stabilizers, in the treatment of bipolar disorder. Moreover, they are also used as adjuncts in the treatment of treatment-resistant major depressive disorder.

Anxiety Screener (GAD-7)

The Generalized Anxiety Disorder 7 (GAD-7) is a self-reported questionnaire for screening and severity measuring of generalized anxiety disorder (GAD). The GAD-7 is normally used in outpatient and primary care settings for referral to a psychiatrist pending outcome.

Adjusted Odds Ratio (AOR)

This is an odds ratio that controls for other predictor variables in a model. It provides an idea of the dynamics between the predictors. Multiple regression, which works with several independent variables, produces AORs.

Arm Design Test (Single and Double)

A single-arm design tests the null hypothesis that the response rate of a new drug is lower than a fixed threshold, whereas a double-arm scheme takes a more objective comparison of the response rate between the new treatment and the standard of care through randomization.

Australian Institute of Health and Welfare Ethics Committee (AIHWEC)

AHEC's composition is specified in the NHMRC Act. Members draw on expertise in philosophy, the ethics of medical research, public health and social science research, clinical medical practice and nursing, disability, law, religion and health consumer issues.

Biennial Faecal Immunochemical testing (BFI)

Fecal Immunochemical Test (FIT) is a diagnostic technique that examines stool samples for traces of non-visible blood, which could potentially indicate conditions including bowel cancer. Symptoms which could be caused by bowel cancer and suggest a FIT include a change in bowel habit, anemia, unexplained weight loss, and abdominal pain.

Binomial Logistic Regression (BLR)

Binomial regression is a regression analysis technique in which the response (often referred to as Y) has a binomial distribution: it is the number of successes in a series of independent Bernoulli trials, where each trial has probability of success p. In binomial regression, the probability of a success is related to explanatory variables: the corresponding concept in ordinary regression is to relate the mean value of the unobserved response to explanatory variables.

Bipolar Disorder (BD)

Previously called manic depression or manic-depressive illness, bipolar disorder (BD) is a serious mental health condition that leads to shifts in mood. It consists of depressive states as well as episodes of mania. During manic episodes, people feel as if they are on a "high" and have extreme amounts of energy.

Black Lion Specialized Hospital, School of Medicine, College of Health Sciences, Addis Ababa University

This is the largest referral hospital in Ethiopia. It was established in 1964, and is now the main teaching center for both clinical and preclinical training of most disciplines. It is also an institution where specialized clinical services that are not available in other public or private institutions are rendered to the whole nation.

BRCA gene test

This test looks for DNA changes that increase the risk of breast cancer and ovarian cancer. BRCA1 and BRCA2 are the most well-known genes. Testing often looks for those genes and many other genes that increase the risk of breast and ovarian cancers.

Breast Cancer Association Consortium (BCAC)

The Breast Cancer Association Consortium (BCAC) is a forum of investigators interested in the inherited risk of breast cancer. Many groups are conducting studies with the aim of identifying genes that may be related to the risk of breast cancer. The aim of the consortium is to combine data from many studies, and to provide a reliable assessment of the risks associated with these genes.

Bridge intervention

This is a person-centered collaborative care model of early integrated psychiatric and cancer care for patients with serious mental illness which was developed to improve cancer outcomes in this underserved population.

Brief Psychiatric Rating Scale (BPRS)

The BPRS assesses the level of 18 symptom constructs such as hostility, suspiciousness, hallucination, and grandiosity. Persons having or suspected of having schizophrenia or other psychotic disorder manifest the disorder in multiple ways. It is particularly useful in gauging the efficacy of treatment in patients who have moderate to severe psychoses.

California Health Interview Survey (CHIS)

The California Health Interview Survey (CHIS) is the nation's largest State health survey and a critical source of data on Californians, as well as on the State's various racial and ethnic groups.

California Medicaid Administrative Records (CMAR)

The California Medical Assistance Program (Medi-Cal or MediCal) is the California implementation of the federal Medicaid program serving low-income individuals, including families, seniors, persons with disabilities, children in foster care, pregnant women, and childless adults with incomes below 138% of federal poverty level.

Cancer Survivor

The American Cancer Society uses the term cancer survivor to refer to anyone who has ever been diagnosed with cancer no matter where they are in the course of their disease.

Case Register Linkage (CRL)

A certificate revocation list (or CRL) is a list of digital certificates that have been revoked by the issuing certificate authority (CA) before their scheduled expiration date and should no longer be trusted.

Charlson Comorbidity Index (CCI)

In medicine, the Charlson Comorbidity Index (CCI) predicts the mortality for a patient who may have a range of concurrent conditions (comorbidities), such as heart disease, AIDS, or cancer (considering a total of 17 categories).

CINAHL

CINAHL stands for the Cumulative Index to Nursing and Allied Health Literature, and the CINAHL Complete database searches for articles in hundreds of nursing journals. In addition to journal articles, researches can find evidence-based care sheets, quick lessons, legal cases, clinical trials, and more.

Clinical Practice Research Datalink (CPRD)

Clinical Practice Research Datalink (CPRD) is a real-world research service supporting retrospective and prospective public health and clinical studies. CPRD research data services are delivered by the Medicines and Healthcare products Regulatory Agency with support from the National Institute for Health and Care Research (NIHR), as part of the Department of Health and Social Care.

Cochrane Library

Cochrane Library (named after Archie Cochrane) is a collection of databases in medicine and other healthcare specialties provided by Cochrane and other organizations. At its core is the collection of Cochrane Reviews, a database of systematic reviews and meta-analyses which summarize and interpret the results of medical research. The Cochrane Library aims to make the results of well-conducted controlled trials readily available and is a key resource in evidence-based medicine.

Colorectal Cancer (CRC)

Colorectal cancer, or CRC, is a disease of the colon or rectum, which are parts of the digestive system. Unlike most cancers, colorectal cancer is often preventable with screening and is highly treatable when detected early.

Common Mental Disorders (CMDs)

Common Mental Disorders (CMDs) refer to depressive and anxiety disorders and are distinct from the feeling of sadness, stress or fear that anyone can experience at some moment in life.

Comorbidity

In the field of medicine, comorbidity is the presence of one or more additional conditions often co-occurring (that is, concomitant or concurrent) with a primary condition. Comorbidity describes the effect of all other conditions an individual patient might have other than the primary condition of interest, and can be physiological or psychological. In the context of mental health, comorbidity often refers to disorders that are often coexistent with each other, such as depression and anxiety disorders.

Complete Mental Health (CMH)

Complete mental health as the presence of social, behavioral, and emotional well-being and resilience factors, as well as minimal social, behavioral, and emotional problems, and the reduction of risk factors.

Composite International Diagnostic Interview for Oncology (CIDI-O)

The CIDI consists of a series of structured modules that screen for somatoform disorders, anxiety, depression, mania, schizophrenia, eating disorders, impairments in cognition, and substance use disorders.

Confidence Intervals (CIs)

A confidence interval (CI) is a range of estimates for an unknown parameter. A confidence interval is computed at a designated *confidence level*; the 95% confidence level is most common, but other levels, such as 90% or 99%, are sometimes used.

Confounding

This term is a distortion (inaccuracy) in the estimated measure of association that occurs when the primary exposure of interest is mixed up with some other factor that is associated with the outcome. Confounding occurs when a competing cause of illness is associated with one or more of the factors being examined under the study hypothesis.

Consultation-Liaison Psychiatry (or consultative psychiatry) (CLP)

This is the branch of psychiatry that specializes in the interface between general medicine/pediatrics and psychiatry, usually taking place in a hospital or medical setting. The role of the consultation-liaison psychiatrist is to see patients with comorbid medical conditions at the request of the treating medical or surgical consultant or team. Consultation-liaison psychiatry has areas of overlap with other disciplines including psychosomatic medicine, health psychology and neuropsychiatry.

Cox Proportional Hazard Models (CPHM)

The purpose of this model is to evaluate simultaneously the effect of several factors on survival. In other words, it allows one to examine how specified factors influence the rate of a particular event happening (e.g., infection, death) at a particular point in time.

Decision-Making Capacity (DMC)

Decision-making capacity (DMC) plays an important role in clinical practice—determining, on the basis of a patient's decisional abilities, whether they are entitled to make their own medical decisions or whether a surrogate must be secured to participate in decisions on their behalf.

De-Identified Data (DID)

This term describes records that have a re-identification code and have enough personally identifiable information removed or obscured so that the remaining information does not identify an individual and there is no reasonable basis to believe that the information can be used to identify a particular individual.

Demoralization

This refers to a state in which there is a perceived inability to cope, that is associated with a sense of disheartenment and a loss of hope and meaning.

Demoralization Scale (DS)

Items are rated on a 5-point Likert scale ranging from 0 (never) to 4 (all the time). A total score for demoralization is calculated by summarizing the single subscale scores. Higher scores indicate higher levels of demoralization.

Depression Screener (PHQ-9)

The PHQ-9 is a multipurpose instrument for screening, diagnosing, monitoring and measuring the severity of depression: The PHQ-9 incorporates DSM-IV depression diagnostic criteria with other leading major depressive symptoms into a brief self-report tool.

Dignity Therapy (DT) narratives

Dignity Therapy (DT) is a brief, individualized, narrative psychotherapy developed to reduce psychosocial and existential distress, and promote dignity, meaning, and hope in end of life patients.

DSM-IV

The *Diagnostic and Statistical Manual of Mental Disorders*, Fourth Edition—DSM-IV—is the official manual of the American Psychiatric Association. Its purpose is to provide a framework for classifying disorders and defining diagnostic criteria for the disorders listed.

DSM-V

The *Diagnostic and Statistical Manual of Mental Disorders*, Fifth Edition, Text Revision (DSM-5-TR) features the most current text updates based on scientific literature with contributions from more than 200 subject matter experts. The substance use disorder criterion of legal problems from the DSM-IV was dropped in favor of cravings or a strong desire or urge to use a substance in the DSM-5. In addition, three categories of disorder severity were formed, using the number of patient symptoms.

EMBASE

Embase (often styled EMBASE for Excerpta Medica dataBASE) is a biomedical and pharmacological bibliographic database of published literature designed to support information managers and pharmacovigilance in complying with the regulatory requirements of a licensed drug. Embase, produced by Elsevier, contains over 32 million records from over 8,500 currently published journals from 1947 to the present.

Endocrine Therapy (ET)

Some breast cancers use the hormone oestrogen in the body to help them grow. Hormone therapy is a treatment that stops the effect of oestrogen on breast cancer cells . Different hormone therapy drugs do this in different ways. Hormone therapy is also sometimes called endocrine therapy.

End of Life (EOL)

This constitutes a recording of cancer patients who have a measurable concern or anxiety regarding issues related to their mortality.

Enhanced Usual Care (EUC)

In an enhanced usual care (EUC) condition, usual care is systematically improved by the research protocol to overcome ethical or methodological problems that would accompany ordinary UC. The degree of enhancement can range from minimal to extensive.

Epithelium

The epithelial tissue is a thin, continuous, protective layer of compactly packed cells with a little intercellular matrix. Epithelial tissues line the outer surfaces of organs and blood vessels throughout the body, as well as the inner surfaces of cavities in many internal organs.

Estrogen receptor (ER) positive.

The cells of this type of breast cancer have receptors that allow them to use the hormone estrogen to grow. Treatment with anti-estrogen hormone (endocrine) therapy can block the growth of the cancer cells.

Euthanasia (EU)

Euthanasia is the practice of ending the life of a patient to limit the patient's suffering. The patient in question would typically be terminally ill or experiencing great pain and suffering. The word “euthanasia” itself comes from the Greek words “eu” (good) and “thanatos” (death).

Fecal Immunochemical Testing (FIT)

FIT (Fecal Immunochemical Test) is a test that looks for blood in a sample of one’s feces. It looks for tiny traces of blood that might not be visually detectable and which could be a sign of cancer. Traces of blood in feces can be caused by other medical conditions and does not necessarily mean you have cancer.

fecal occult blood testing (gFOBT)

This test looks at a sample of one’s feces to check for blood. Occult blood means that you can't see it with the naked eye. Blood in the stool means there is bleeding in the digestive tract.

Finnish Cancer Registry (FCR)

The Finnish Cancer Registry maintains the national registry of all the diagnosed cancer cases since 1953. It is also a statistical and epidemiological research institute that does active collaboration both nationally and internationally.

Finnish Hospital Discharge Register (FHDR)

The Finnish Hospital Discharge Register (FHDR) is one of the oldest individual level hospital discharge registers and has been intensively used for research purposes. The aim of this study was to gather information concerning the quality of FHDR into one place in terms of a systematic review of validation studies that compare data to external information.

Generic Inverse Variance Method (GIVM)

In the inverse variance method the weight given to each study is the inverse of the variance of the effect estimate (i.e. one over the square of its standard error). Thus larger studies are given more weight than smaller studies, which have larger standard errors.

guaiac Fecal Occult Blood Testing (gFOBT)

This test can detect small amounts of blood in stool. It requires abstaining from red meat and certain medications for a number of days before. An FOBT is more specific to finding blood from further up the digestive tract, such as the stomach.

Guideline-Concordant Treatment (GCT)

This is defined as the minimal treatment patients should receive according to the National Comprehensive Cancer Network guidelines.

Hazard ratio (HR)

In survival analysis, the hazard ratio is the ratio of the hazard rates corresponding to the conditions characterised by two distinct levels of a treatment variable of interest. For example, in a clinical study of a drug, the treated population may die at twice the rate per unit time of the control population.

Head and Neck Cancer (HNC)

Head and neck cancer (HNC) is a group of epithelial malignancies involving the upper shared respiratory/digestive tract (lips, oral cavity, oropharynx, nasal cavity, nasopharynx, hypopharynx and larynx/upper trachea), the salivary glands and lymphadenopathy associated with these diseases.

Hereditary Breast and Ovarian Cancer (HBOC)

Hereditary Breast and Ovarian Cancer syndrome (HBOC) is a genetic condition that makes it more likely that a person will get breast, ovarian, and other cancers. HBOC is hereditary, meaning that it is caused by a mutation (genetic change) that can be passed down in families.

High-Grade Precancerous Cervical Lesions (CIN2+)

The cervical dysplasia is moderate to severe and the cells are considered more abnormal. With HSIL, there are distinct changes to the size and shape of the cells so they look different from normal cells. CIN 2 is moderate to severe dysplasia. CIN 3 is severe dysplasia and also includes carcinoma in *situ*.

Hospital Discharge Register (HDR)

National Hospital Discharge Register (HDR) has been maintained from 1967 in Finland. Clinicians assign diagnoses and ICD codes for every hospitalized patient and codes are then recorded to HDR. HDR is maintained by the National Institute of Health and Welfare.

HPSA Care Shortage Status

Health Professional Shortage Area (HPSA) designations are used to identify areas and population groups within the United States that are experiencing a shortage of health professionals.

HPV vaccine

Human papillomavirus vaccines are vaccines that prevent infection by certain types of human papillomavirus. Available HPV vaccines protect against either two, four, or nine types of HPV. All HPV vaccines protect against at least HPV types 16 and 18, which cause the greatest risk of cervical cancer.

Human Epidermal Growth Factor Receptor 2 (HER2)

Human papillomavirus vaccines are vaccines that prevent infection by certain types of human papillomavirus. Available HPV vaccines protect against either two, four, or nine types of HPV. All HPV vaccines protect against at least HPV types 16 and 18, which cause the greatest risk of cervical cancer.

Hyperprolactinemia

This is marked by abnormally high levels of the hormone prolactin (which stimulates breast milk production during and after pregnancy) in the blood. It is caused by a benign tumor (prolactoma) in the pituitary gland, which controls production of this hormone.

ICD9/10CM code (Mental illness classification)

Mental, Behavioral and Neurodevelopmental disorders ICD-10-CM Code range F01-F99. The ICD-10 code range for

Mental, Behavioral and Neurodevelopmental disorders F01-F99 and is medical classification list by the World Health Organization (WHO).

ICES (formerly known as the Institute for Clinical Evaluative Sciences)

This is an independent, non-profit corporation that applies the study of health informatics for health services research and population-wide health outcomes research in Ontario, Canada, using data collected through the routine administration of Ontario's system of publicly funded health care.

Incidence Rate Ratios (IRR)

An incidence rate ratio (IRR) is a meaningful effect measure in epidemiology if it is adjusted for all important confounders. For evaluation of the impact of adjustment, adjusted IRRs should be compared with crude IRRs.

International Classification of Diseases (ICD)

The International Classification of Diseases is a globally used medical classification used in epidemiology, health management and for clinical purposes. The ICD is maintained by the World Health Organization, which is the directing and coordinating authority for health within the United Nations System.

International Prostate Symptom Score (IPSS)

The International Prostate Symptom Score (IPSS) is an eight-question written screening tool used to screen for, rapidly diagnose, track the symptoms of, and suggest management of the lower urinary tract symptoms of benign prostatic hyperplasia (BPH).

IPOS Standards of Quality Cancer Care

IPOS International Standard of Quality Cancer Care Quality cancer care must integrate the psychosocial domain into routine care; Distress should be measured as the 6th Vital Sign after temperature, blood pressure, pulse, respiratory rate and pain.

Irremediability of a Mental Disorder (IMD)

A mental disorder which cannot be treated with measurable success over time with treatment modalities currently employed by the health care community.

Kessler K6 Screening Tool (KK6S)

The Kessler Psychological Distress Scale (K6+) is a 6-item self-report measure of psychological distress intended to be used as a quick tool to assess risk for serious mental illness in the general population.

Kessler Nonspecific Mental/Psychological Distress Scale (KNMPDS)

The Kessler Psychological Distress Scale (K10) is a simple measure of psychological distress. The K10 scale involves 10 questions about emotional states each with a five-level response scale. The measure can be used as a brief screen to identify levels of distress.

Latent Class Analyses (LCA)

Latent class analysis (LCA) is the label given to a form of finite mixture modeling where the observed indicators are all categorical. Latent Profile Analysis is the term used for mixture modelling where the indicators are all numerical and continuous in their distribution.

Likert scale

This is a type of rating scale, often found on survey forms or questionnaires, that measures how people feel and levels of agreement which can be useful in many different situations.

Long-Term Condition (LTC)

This is a medical condition that generally lasts a year or longer and impacts a person's life. Examples include arthritis, asthma, cancer, dementia, diabetes, heart disease, mental health conditions and stroke. Long-term conditions may also be known as 'chronic conditions'.

Low- and Lower-Middle-Income Countries (LLMICs)

For the current 2024 fiscal year, low-income economies are defined as those with a GNI per capita, calculated using the World Bank Atlas method, of $1,135 or less in 2022; lower middle-income economies are those with a GNI per capita between $1,136 and $4,465.

Lung Cancer Screening (LCS)

Lung cancer screening refers to cancer screening strategies used to identify early lung cancers before they cause symptoms, at a point where they are more likely to be curable. Lung cancer screening is critically important because of the incidence and prevalence of lung cancer.

Major Depressive Disorder (MDD)

Major depressive disorder (MDD) has been ranked as the third cause of the burden of disease worldwide in 2008 by WHO, which has projected that this disease will rank first by 2030. It is diagnosed when an individual has a persistently low or depressed mood, anhedonia or decreased interest in pleasurable activities, feelings of guilt or worthlessness, lack of energy, poor concentration, appetite changes, psychomotor retardation or agitation, sleep disturbances, or suicidal thoughts.

Mantel-Haenszel Approach (MHA)

The Cochran-Mantel-Haenszel method is a technique that generates an estimate of an association between an exposure and an outcome after adjusting for or taking into account confounding. The method is used with a dichotomous outcome variable and a dichotomous risk factor.

Mastectomy

This is a surgery to remove a breast. Sometimes other tissues near the breast, such as lymph nodes, are also removed. This surgery is most often used to treat breast cancer. In some cases, a mastectomy is done to help prevent breast cancer in women who have a high risk for it.

MarketScan (MS)

The IBM® MarketScan® Commercial Database consists of medical and drug data from employers and health plans. It contains data for several million individuals annually, encompassing employees, their spouses and dependents who are covered by employer- sponsored private health insurance in the US.

Matched Cohort

This study involves pairs (or clusters in case several untreated subjects are matched with each of the treated individuals) formed to include individuals who differ with respect to treatment but may be matched on certain baseline characteristics.

Medical Assistance in Dying (MAiD)

Medical aid in dying (MAID) is a practice in which a physician provides a competent adult with a terminal illness with a prescription for a lethal dose of a drug at the request of the patient, which the patient intends to use to end his or her life.

MEDLine

MEDLINE (Medical Literature Analysis and Retrieval System Online, or MEDLARS Online) is a bibliographic database of life sciences and biomedical information. It includes bibliographic information for articles from academic journals covering medicine, nursing, pharmacy, dentistry, veterinary medicine, and health care. MEDLINE also covers much of the literature in biology and biochemistry, as well as fields such as molecular evolution.

Mendelian Randomization (MR) research

Mendelian randomization is a method of using measured variation in genes of known function to examine the causal effect of a modifiable exposure on disease in observational studies.

Mental Disorders (MDs) (aka mental illness, psychiatric disorders)

These are defined as health conditions that affect and alter cognitive functioning, emotional responses, and behavior associated with distress and/or impaired functioning. The ICD-11 is the global standard used to diagnose, treat, research, and report various mental disorders.

Mental Health Disorder (MHD)

Related to Mental Health Division. Mental health services means interventions designed to provide the maximum reduction of mental disability and restoration or maintenance of functioning consistent with the requirements for learning, development and enhanced self-sufficiency.

Mental Health Research Network (MHRN)

Since 2010, the Mental Health Research Network (MHRN) has sought to improve population mental health and the delivery of mental health care. With 14 member research centers and partner health systems, the MHRN has the ability to carry out population-based mental health research with unprecedented scale and efficiency.

Mental Health Services (MHS)

Managed Health Services (MHS) is a health insurance provider that has been proudly serving Indiana residents for more than twenty-five years through Hoosier Healthwise, the Healthy Indiana Plan (HIP) and Hoosier Care Connect.

Meta-analysis

This is a quantitative, formal, epidemiological study design used to systematically assess the results of previous research to derive conclusions about that body of research.

Typically, but not necessarily, the study is based on randomized, controlled clinical trials.

Ministry of Health and Welfare Data Science Center (MHWDSC)

The National Health Insurance system of Taiwan was established in 1995 and covers more than 99.6% of the Taiwanese population; this system's claims data are released as the National Health Insurance Research Database (NHIRD). All data from primary outpatient departments and inpatient hospital care settings after 2000 are included in this database.

Mortality Rate Ratios (MRR)

MRRs: Represent the ratio of mortality rates between persons with and without a diagnosis of the specific disorder adjusted for age, sex, and birth date.

National Bowel Cancer Screening Programme (NBCSP)

National Bowel Cancer Screening Program is an initiative by the Federal Government that aims to reduce death from bowel cancer through early detection.

National Epidemiologic Survey on Alcohol and Related Conditions (NESARC)

The National Epidemiologic Study of Alcohol Related Conditions (NESARC) is a random sample survey of the United States population conducted in two waves by researchers at the Laboratory of Epidemiology and Biometry of the National Institute on Alcohol Abuse and Alco- holism (NIAAA).

National Health Interview Surveys (NHIS)

The main objective of the National Health Interview Survey (NHIS) is to monitor the health of the United States population through collection and analysis of data on a broad range of health topics.

National Health Service Breast Screening Programme (NHSBSP)

The NHS Breast Screening Programme invites all women from the age of 50 to 70 registered with a GP for screening every 3 years. This means that some people may not have their first screening mammogram until they are 52 or 53 years.

Nationwide Readmissions Database (NRD)

The Nationwide Readmissions Database (NRD) is a unique and powerful database designed to support various types of analyses of national readmissions for all patients regardless of the expected payer for the hospital stay.

Neo-Plasm Staging

This is the process of finding out how much cancer is in a person's body and where it's located. It's how the doctor determines the stage of a person's cancer.

Nested Case–Control Study

This is a variation of a case–control study in which cases and controls are drawn from the population in a fully enumerated cohort. Usually, the exposure of interest is only measured among the cases and the selected controls.

Newcastle-Ottawa scale

The Newcastle-Ottawa Scale (NOS) is a validated, easy to use scale of 8 items in three domains, selection, comparability, and outcome. The NOS is used to assess the quality of the included studies.

New York State Cancer Registry (NYSCR)

The NYSCR is a population-based cancer incidence registry responsible for the collection of demographic, diagnostic and treatment information on all patients diagnosed with and/or treated for cancer at hospitals, laboratories, and other health care facilities throughout New York State.

Northern Ireland Longitudinal Study (NILS)

The Northern Ireland Longitudinal Study (NILS) has been formally available to researchers since the end of 2006. It comprises two major data linkage studies: the NILS and the Northern Ireland Mortality Study (NIMS). These were developed by NISRA and are maintained and managed by them as a resource for research.

Nosological Systems

The nosological diagnosis is a particular type of nontheoretical diagnosis consisting of identifying the disease that afflicts the patient without explaining the underlying etiopathological mechanisms.

Nulliparous

This is a medical term used to describe a woman who has not given birth to a child. It doesn't necessarily mean that she's never been pregnant — someone who's had a miscarriage, stillbirth, or elective abortion but has never given birth to a live baby is still referred to as nulliparous.

Odds Ratios (OR)

The odds ratio (OR) is a measure of how strongly an event is associated with exposure. The odds ratio is a ratio of two sets of odds: the odds of the event occurring in an exposed group versus the odds of the event occurring in a non-exposed group. Odds ratios commonly are used to report case-control studies.

Otolaryngology

This is a medical specialty which is focused on the ears, nose, and throat. It is also called otolaryngology-head and neck surgery because specialists are trained in both medicine and surgery. An otolaryngologist is often called an ear, nose, and throat doctor, or an ENT for short.

OVID

Ovid is the world's leading information search, discovery, and management solution providing professionals in science, medicine, and healthcare with a single online destination for accessing premium journals, books and databases.

Partial Laryngectomy (PRL)

A partial laryngectomy is the surgical removal of a portion of the larynx, or the voice box. This procedure is usually done for patients with cancer of the larynx. A partial laryngectomy may be possible versus a total laryngectomy, depending on the extent of the cancer. With the partial laryngectomy you may retain some normal speech and more of your normal swallowing function.

Patient Health Questionnaire-9 (PHQ-9)

The Patient Health Questionnaire (PHQ) is a self-administered version of the PRIME-MD diagnostic instrument for common mental disorders. The PHQ-9 is the depression module, which scores each of the 9 DSM-IV criteria as "0" (not at all) to "3" (nearly every day).

Person Centered Cancer Screening Services (PECCS)

Person Centered Cancer Screening (PECCS) research study, investigating how cancer screening services can be changed to help people with learning disabilities and/or severe mental illness.

Physician-Assisted Death/Suicide (PAD/S)

Physician-Assisted Dying (PAD) is defined as a physician providing, at the patient's request, a prescription for a lethal dose of medication that the patient can self-administer by ingestion, with the explicit intention of ending life.

Poisson Models (PMs)

The Poisson model is a discrete probability distribution that expresses the probability of a number of events occurring in a fixed period of time (but also in other specified intervals such as distance or area) if these events occur with a known average rate and independently of the time since the last event.

Polycystic Ovary Syndrome (PCOS)

Polycystic ovary syndrome (PCOS) is a condition in which the ovaries produce an abnormal amount of androgens, male sex hormones that are usually present in women in small amounts. The name polycystic ovary syndrome describes the numerous small cysts (fluid-filled sacs) that form in the ovaries.

Post-Traumatic Stress/Adjustment Disorder (PTSD/AD)

An adjustment disorder is a strong emotional or behavioral reaction to stress or trauma. It causes short-term symptoms that may make one react more than one typically would. One may cry easily or feel depressed and hopeless. One might overindulge in risky behaviors, or act recklessly or impulsively.

Partial laryngectomy (PRL)

This is the surgical removal of a portion of the larynx, or the voice box. This procedure is usually done for patients with cancer of the larynx.

Precancerous Cervical Lesions (CIN2)

This is not cancer but may become cancer and spread to nearby normal tissue if not treated. Treatment for CIN 2 may include cryotherapy, laser therapy, loop electrosurgical procedure (LEEP), or cone biopsy to remove or destroy the abnormal tissue. CIN 2 is sometimes called high-grade or moderate dysplasia.

PRISMA Guidelines

PRISMA stands for Preferred Reporting Items for Systematic Reviews and Meta-Analyses. It is an evidence-based minimum set of items for reporting in systematic reviews and meta-analyses.

PROLACTIN (PRL)

(Also known as lactotropin and PRL) is a hormone that is responsible for lactation, certain breast tissue development and contributes to hundreds of other bodily processes. Prolactin levels are normally low in people assigned male at birth (AMAB) and non-lactating and non-pregnant people.

Progesterone receptor (PR) positive.

This type of breast cancer is sensitive to progesterone, and the cells have receptors that allow them to use this hormone to grow. Treatment with endocrine therapy blocks the growth of cancer cells.

PROSPERO

The International Prospective Register of Systematic Reviews, better known as PROSPERO, is an open access online database of systematic review protocols on a wide range of topics. While it was initially restricted to medicine, as of 2021, it also accepts protocols in criminology, social care, education and international development, as long as there is a health-related outcome. Researchers can choose to have their reviews prospectively registered with PROSPERO.

PsychInfo

APA PsycInfo is an abstracts database that provides systematic coverage of the psychological literature from the 1800s to the present. (The database also includes some records from the 1600s and 1700s.)

Psychotropic medication

A psychoactive drug, psychopharmaceutical, psychoactive agent, or psychotropic drug is a chemical substance that changes the function of the nervous system and results in alterations of perception, mood, cognition, and behavior.

PsycLIT

PsycLIT contained citations and abstracts to journal articles, and summaries of English-language chapters and books in psychology, as well as behavioral information from sociology, linguistics, medicine, law, psychiatry, and anthropology.

PubMed

PubMed is a free resource supporting the search and retrieval of biomedical and life sciences literature with the aim of improving health–both globally and personally. The PubMed database contains more than 36 million citations and abstracts of biomedical literature.

Psychiatric Genomics Consortium (PGC)

The Psychiatric Genomics Consortium (PGC) is an international consortium of scientists dedicated to conducting meta- and mega-analyses of genomic-wide genetic data, with a focus on psychiatric disorders.

Radical Cystectomy

This procedure is used to remove the entire bladder. In men, this typically includes removal of the prostate and seminal vesicles. In women, radical cystectomy usually includes removal of the uterus, ovaries, fallopian tubes and part of the vagina.

Randomized Controlled Trials (RCTs)

Randomized controlled trials (RCT) are prospective studies that measure the effectiveness of a new intervention or treatment. Although no study is likely on its own to prove causality, randomization reduces bias and provides a rigorous tool to examine cause-effect relationships between an intervention and outcome.

Research Ethics Committee and Trust Research & Development (RECTRD)

A research ethics committee is a group of people appointed to review research proposals to assess formally if the research is ethical. This means the research must conform to recognized ethical standards, which includes respecting the dignity, rights, safety and well-being of the people who take part.

SCOPUS

Scopus is Elsevier's abstract and citation database launched in 2004. Scopus covers nearly 36,377 titles (22,794 active titles and 13,583 inactive titles) from approximately 11,678 publishers, of which 34,346 are peer-reviewed journals in top-level subject fields: life sciences, social sciences, physical sciences and health sciences. It covers three types of sources: book series, journals, and trade journals.

Sequencing Diagnosis Coding

Medical coders are tasked with selecting the most specific codes and putting them in the right order. This code arrangement is called “sequencing,” and it is an essential step to correct coding.

SEER-Medicare database

The SEER-Medicare data reflect the linkage of two large population-based sources of data that provide detailed information about elderly persons with cancer, which can be used for an array of epidemiological and health services research.

Self-Reporting Questionnaire (SRQ-20)

The 20-item Self Reporting Questionnaire (SRQ-20) was developed to screen for non-psychotic disorders. It consists of 20 yes/no questions asking respondents about symptoms and problems likely to occur in people with neurotic disorders in the past 30 days.

Serious Mental Illness (SrMI or SMI)

The research is inconsistent in its use of the terms "serious" and "severe" such that the psychotherapeutic community along with the psychiatric community has chosen at this point not to make a clinical distinction between the terms. Therefore and in spite of the ambiguity of use, *serious mental illness* and *severe mental illness* are still correctly used interchangeably.

Severe and Persistent Mental Illness (SPMI)

Severe persistent mental illnesses (SPMIs) are those that are prolonged and recurrent, impair activities of daily living, and require long-term treatment. Common diagnoses include schizophrenia, bipolar disorder, and major depression.

Severe Mental Illness (SvMI or SMI) (such as schizophrenia and severe mood disorders)

Severe Mental Illness (SMI) – SMI is a smaller and more severe subset of mental illnesses; SMI is defined as one or more mental, behavioral, or emotional disorder(s) resulting in serious functional impairment, which substantially interferes with or limits one or more major life activities (NIMH). Schizophrenia and bi-polar disorder are the most common illness in SMI.

Severe Psychiatric Illness (SPI)

SPI includes major depression, schizophrenia, bipolar disorder, obsessive compulsive disorder (OCD), panic disorder, post-traumatic stress (PTSD) and borderline personality disorder (VA).

Shared decision making (SDM)

This is defined as "…a formal process or tool that helps physicians and patients work together to choose the treatment option that best reflects both medical evidence and the individual patient's priorities and goals for his or her care (American Medical Association, 2012)."

Significant Mental Health Difficulties (SMHD)

Mental health includes our emotional, psychological, and social well-being. It affects how we think, feel, and act. It also helps determine how we handle stress, relate to others, and make healthy choices. Mental health is important at every stage of life, from childhood and adolescence through adulthood.

Single Nucleotide Polymorphism (SNP)

Single nucleotide polymorphisms, frequently called SNPs (pronounced "snips"), are the most common type of genetic variation among people. Each SNP represents a difference in a single DNA building block, called a nucleotide.

Spiritual Care

This is an aspect of health care that supports the inner person to help deal with the health challenges that the cancer patients or the patient's loved one is facing. This may include concerns or questions about personal meaning, purpose, legacy, hope and faith. Because cancer patients cover the gambit of intense religious faith to no faith at all, spiritual care is not predicated upon a belief in a Transcendent Reality but rather focuses upon the patient's own sense of the meaning and purpose of life.

SPSS for Windows, Version 16.0. Chicago, SPSS Inc.

SPSS Statistics is a statistical software suite developed by IBM for data management, advanced analytics, multivariate analysis, business intelligence, and criminal investigation. Long produced by SPSS Inc., it was acquired by IBM in 2009. Versions of the software released since 2015 have the brand name IBM SPSS Statistics.

Standardized Mean Difference (SMD)

Standardized Mean Difference and Cohen's d: Effect Size Measurement. The standardized mean difference (SMD) measure of effect is used when studies report efficacy in terms of a continuous measurement, such as a score on a pain-intensity rating scale. The SMD is also known as Cohen's d.

Structured Clinical Interview for DSM-IV (SCID)

The Structured Clinical Interview for DSM-IV (SCID) is a semi-structured interview created to make reliable psychiatric diagnoses in adults according to the *Diagnostic and Statistical Manual*, fourth edition (DSM-IV).

Suboptimal health status (SHS)

This is defined as a state characterized by some disturbances in psychological behaviors or physical characteristics, or in some indices of medical examination, with no typical pathologic features.

Substance Use Disorder (SUD)

Substance use disorder (SUD) is a treatable mental disorder that affects a person's brain and behavior, leading to their inability to control their use of substances like legal or illegal drugs, alcohol, or medications. Symptoms can be moderate to severe, with addiction being the most severe form of SUD.

Suicidal Ideation (SI)

Suicidal ideations (SI), often called suicidal thoughts or ideas, is a broad term used to describe a range of contemplations, wishes, and preoccupations with death and suicide.

Survival Analysis (SA)

This constitutes a collection of statistical procedures for data analysis where the outcome variable of interest is timed until an event occurs. Because of censoring–the non-observation of the event of interest after a period of follow-up–a proportion of the survival times of interest will often be unknown.

Swedish Patient Register (SPR)

From 1987 SPR includes all in-patient care in Sweden. Since 2001 the register also covers outpatient doctor visits including day surgery and psychiatric care from both private and public caregivers.

Synergistic effects

These are the combined effects of at least two substances making an impact that is more significant than both of them could have shown by themselves. Etymology: from Greek "synergos", meaning "working together".

Ten-Item Personality Inventory (TIPI)

The Ten-Item Personality Inventory (TIPI) is a brief assessment of the Big Five personality dimensions: (1) Extraversion, (2) Agreeableness, (3) Conscientiousness, (4) Emotional Stability, and (5) Openness to Experience. Items are rated on a scale from 1, disagree strongly, to 7, agree strongly.

Transoral Surgery (TS)

Transoral robotic surgery is a type of operation that uses a computer system to help guide the surgical tools. The tools are passed through the mouth to access the mouth and throat. Transoral robotic surgery is one option for treating mouth cancer and throat cancer.

Trimodal Therapy (TT)

This involves having a shorter time-frame for surgery to remove the tumour from the bladder (TURBT), followed by radiation therapy combined with chemotherapy (chemoradiation). Some people who are not fit enough for chemotherapy will have radiation therapy on its own.

University of Queensland Human Research Ethics Committee (UQHREC)

The HREC functions on behalf of UQ to: 2.1 Provide independent oversight of human research projects; 2.2 Provide competent, timely review and monitoring of human research projects. in respect of their ethical and scientific acceptability for the length of time required for any project.

Uptake

This is typically defined as the percentage of those individual patients invited who receive an adequate screen (a definitive test result) within a specified period after their test. Uptake has been described as the most important factor in determining the success of a cancer screening program.

Urothelial Carcinoma (also called transitional cell carcinoma) (UC)

This is a type of cancer that begins in the urothelial cells, which line the urethra, bladder, ureters, renal pelvis, and some other organs. Almost all bladder cancers are urothelial carcinomas.

World Health Organization Composite International Diagnostic Interview (WHOCIDI)

The World Health Organization Composite International Diagnostic Interview (CIDI) is a structured interview for psychiatric disorders. As the interview is designed for epidemiological studies, it can be administered by those who are not clinically trained and can be completed in a short period of time.

World Mental Health Surveys (WMHSs)

The World Mental Health (WMH) surveys are a coordinated set of community psychiatric epidemiological surveys conducted in 30 countries to date. The WMH Survey Initiative began as a project of the Assessment, Classification, and Epidemiology (ACE) Group at the World Health Organization coordinating the implementation and analysis of general population epidemiologic surveys of mental, substance use, and behavioral disorders in countries in all WHO Regions.

World Mental Health Survey Initiative (WMHSI)

The WMH Survey Initiative aims to obtain accurate cross-national information about the prevalence and correlates of mental, substance, and behavioral disorders. Included in studies of correlates will be analyses of impairments, other adverse social consequences, and patterns of help-seeking.

**Definitions gleaned and edited from google, wikipedia, and relevant web sites.*

B. PERIODICALS CITED

(Descriptions are based on abridgements from google, wikipedia and the periodical websites.) NOTE: Abbreviations have been retained from the Bibliographic citations.

Acta Oncol Acta Oncologica is a peer-reviewed medical journal of oncology and the official journal of the five Nordic oncological societies. It is published by Taylor and Francis Group and was established in 1963.

Aging Ment Health Aging & Mental Health is a peer-reviewed monthly scientific journal published by Routledge covering research on the relationship between the aging process and mental health.

Am J Clin Oncol.

Am J Health Promot *The American Journal of Health Promotion* (AJHP) is a peer-reviewed journal advancing the science of health behavior change and the art of creating a culture of well-being. Established in 1986.

Am J Prev Med The American Journal of Preventive Medicine is a monthly peer-reviewed medical journal that publishes articles in the areas of prevention research, teaching, practice and policy.

Am J Surg The American Journal of Surgery is a peer-reviewed scientific journal published by Elsevier on behalf of 6 major surgical societies.

Ann Oncol The Annals of Oncology is a peer-reviewed medical journal of oncology, published by Elsevier. It is the official journal of the European Society for Medical Oncology.

Ann Otol Rhinol Laryngol The *Annals of Otology, Rhinology & Laryngology* publishes original manuscripts of clinical and research importance in otolaryngology-head and neck medicine and surgery, bronchoesophagology, head and neck oncology and surgery, plastic and reconstructive surgery, pediatric otolaryngology, audiology, speech pathology, and related specialties.

Arch Gerontol Geriatr *Archives of Gerontology and Geriatrics* provides a medium for the publication of papers from the fields of experimental gerontology and clinical and social geriatrics.

Arch Psychiatr Nurs *Archives of Psychiatric Nursing* disseminates original, peer-reviewed research that is of interest to psychiatric and mental health care nurses. The field is considered in its broadest perspective, including theory, practice and research applications related to all ages.

Aust N Z J Psychiatry Australian and New Zealand Journal of Psychiatry is a peer-reviewed academic journal that publishes papers in the field of Psychiatry.

BMC Cancer BMC Cancer is a peer-reviewed open access medical journal that publishes original research on cancer and oncology. It was established in 2001 at a time when open access publishing was in its infancy.

BMC Health Serv Res BMC Health Services Research is an open access healthcare journal, which covers research on the subject of health services.

BMJ Open BMJ Open is a peer-reviewed open access medical journal that is dedicated to publishing medical research from all disciplines and therapeutic areas.

Breast Cancer Res Treat Breast Cancer Research and Treatment is a scientific journal focused on the treatment of and investigations in breast cancer. It is targeted towards a wide audience of clinical researchers, epidemiologists, immunologists, or cell biologists interested in breast cancer.

Breast Breast is a peer-reviewed medical journal published by Elsevier covering research on breast cancer. It is an associate journal of the Australasian Society for Breast Disease.

Breast J *The Breast* is a multidisciplinary open access journal for researchers and clinicians, which focuses on translational and clinical research for the advancement of breast cancer prevention, diagnosis and treatment of all stages.

Brit J Cancer The British Journal of Cancer is a twice-monthly professional medical journal owned by Cancer Research UK, published on their behalf by Springer Nature's Nature Research.

Br J Psychiatry The British Journal of Psychiatry is a peer-reviewed medical journal covering all branches of psychiatry with a particular emphasis on the clinical aspects of each topic. The journal is owned by the Royal College of Psychiatrists and published monthly by Cambridge University Press on behalf of the college.

CA Cancer J. Clin. CA: A Cancer Journal for Clinicians is a bimonthly peer-reviewed medical journal published for the American Cancer Society by Wiley-Blackwell. The journal was established in 1950 and covers aspects of cancer research on diagnosis, therapy, and prevention.

Cancer Control *Cancer Control* is a JCR-ranked, peer-reviewed open access journal whose mission is to advance the prevention, detection, diagnosis, treatment, and palliative care of cancer by enabling researchers, doctors, policymakers, and other healthcare professionals to freely share research along the cancer control continuum.

Cancer *Cancer*, an international interdisciplinary journal of the American Cancer Society, publishes high-impact, peer-reviewed original articles and solicited content on the latest clinical research findings. Each issue of *Cancer* strives to be comprehensive, spanning the breadth of oncology disciplines and providing something for everyone involved in cancer research, risk reduction, treatment, and patient care.

Cancer Med. *Cancer Medicine* is an open access, interdisciplinary oncology journal providing rapid publication of research from global biomedical researchers across the cancer sciences. Indexed in Medline and Web of Science, we cover the breadth of oncology: clinical cancer research, cancer biology, cancer prevention, and bioinformatics.

Cancer Nurs *Cancer Nursing*™ addresses the whole spectrum of problems arising in the care and support of cancer patients--prevention and early detection, geriatric and pediatric cancer nursing, medical and surgical oncology, ambulatory care, nutritional support, psychosocial aspects of cancer, patient responses to all treatment modalities, and specific nursing interventions. The journal offers unparalleled coverage of cancer care delivery practices worldwide, as well as groundbreaking research findings and their practical applications.

Contemp Clin Trials Contemporary Clinical Trials is a monthly peer-reviewed medical journal covering clinical trials and research design in clinical medicine.

Current Problems in Cancer Current Problems in Cancer seeks to promote and disseminate innovative, transformative, and impactful data on patient-oriented cancer research and clinical care. Specifically, the journal's scope is focused on reporting the results of well-designed cancer studies.

Dig Dis Sci Digestive Diseases and Sciences, formerly known as the American Journal of Digestive Diseases, is a monthly peer-reviewed journal focusing on gastroenterology and hepatology.

Epidemiol Psychiatr Sci Epidemiology and Psychiatric Sciences is a quarterly peer-reviewed scientific journal covering psychiatry and epidemiology.

Eur Arch Otorhinolaryngol European Archives of Oto-Rhino-Laryngology publishes original clinical reports and clinically relevant experimental studies, as well as short communications presenting new results of special interest. With peer review by a respected international editorial board and prompt English-language publication, the journal provides rapid dissemination of information by authors from around the world.

Eur J Cancer The European Journal of Cancer is a peer-reviewed medical journal devoted to cancer research on experimental oncology, clinical oncology, and on cancer epidemiology and prevention.

Eur Rev Med Pharmacol Sci European Review for Medical and Pharmacological Sciences, a fortnightly journal, acts as an information exchange tool on several aspects of medical and pharmacological sciences. It publishes reviews, original articles, and results from original research.

Eur Urol Focus *European Urology Focus* (EU Focus) is to encompass the whole spectrum of urology. The journal publishes papers on a wide range of urological issues such as oncology, functional urology, reconstructive urology, laparoscopy, robotic surgery, endourology, female urology, andrology, paediatric urology and sexual medicine. The editorial team welcomes basic and translational research articles in the field of urological diseases.

Gen Hosp Psychiatry *General Hospital Psychiatry* explores the many linkages among psychiatry, medicine, and primary care. In emphasizing a biopsychosocial approach to illness and health, the journal provides a forum for professionals with clinical, academic, and research interests in psychiatry's role.

HPB (Oxford) *HPB* is an international forum for clinical, scientific and educational communication. Twelve issues a year bring the reader leading articles, expert reviews, original articles, images, editorials, and reader correspondence encompassing all aspects of benign and malignant hepatobiliary disease and its management. *HPB* features relevant aspects of clinical and translational research and practice.

Int J Clin Pract The International Journal of Clinical Practice is a monthly peer-reviewed general medical journal.

International Journal of Psychiatry in Medicine The goal of *The International Journal of Psychiatry in Medicine* is to address the complex relationships among biological, psychological, social, religious and cultural systems in patient care.

Int Rev Psychiatry *The International Review of Psychiatry* is the premier review journal in the field with a truly international authorship and readership. Each bimonthly issue is dedicated to a specific theme relevant to psychiatry, edited by recognized experts on the topic.

J. Adv. Nurs The Journal of Advanced Nursing is a monthly peer-reviewed medical journal covering all aspects of nursing.

JAMA Oncol JAMA Oncology is a monthly peer-reviewed medical journal published by the American Medical

Association. It covers all aspects of medical oncology, radiation oncology, and surgical oncology, as well as subspecialties.

JAMA Otolaryngol Head Neck Surg *JAMA Otolaryngology—Head & Neck Surgery* is a monthly peer-reviewed medical journal published by the American Medical Association and covering all aspects of prevention, diagnosis, and treatment of diseases of the head, neck, ear, nose, and throat.

J Am Coll Radiol The Journal of the American College of Radiology is a monthly peer-reviewed medical journal covering radiology.

J Anxiety Disord Journal of Anxiety Disorders is a bimonthly peer-reviewed interdisciplinary academic journal publishing research on all aspects of anxiety disorders across the lifespan.

J Cancer Res Ther The *Journal of Cancer Research and Therapeutics* is a peer-reviewed open access medical journal published on behalf of the Association of Radiation Oncologists of India. The journal covers research in oncology, radiation oncology, medical imaging, radiation protection, non-ionising radiation, and radiobiology.

J Clin Oncol The *Journal of Clinical Oncology* is a peer-reviewed medical journal published 3 times a month by the Lippincott Williams & Wilkins. It covers research on all aspects of clinical oncology.

J Psychosom Res The *Journal of Psychiatric Research* is a monthly peer-reviewed medical journal covering research in four major areas of psychiatry: clinical studies on normal and pathological human behavior; basic studies in psychiatry and related fields; clinical laboratory techniques such as neuroimaging, spectroscopy and other computer techniques used in research; advances in research methodology, including the clinical use of recent research findings.

JCO Oncol Pract JCO Oncology Practice is a monthly peer-reviewed medical journal covering the mechanics of oncology care. It was established in 2005 and is published by the American Society of Clinical Oncology.

J Dual Diagn *Journal of Dual Diagnosis* is a quarterly, international publication that focuses on the full spectrum of complexities regarding dual diagnosis. The co-occurrence of mental health and substance use disorders, or "dual diagnosis," is one of the quintessential issues in behavioral health.

J Epidemiol Community Health The Journal of Epidemiology and Community Health is a monthly peer-reviewed public health journal that covers all aspects of epidemiology and public health.

J Med Imaging Radiat Sci The *Journal of Medical Imaging and Radiation Sciences (JMIRS)* is the official bilingual, peer-reviewed journal of the Canadian Association of Medical Radiation Technologists (CAMRT) and international associations across four continents, including the Hong Kong Radiographers Association (HKRA); Portuguese Association of Nuclear Medicine Technologists (APTMN); Alliance In Nuclear Scintigraphy (RAINS) in Australia; and Society of Medical Radiographers - Malta.

J Obstet Gynaecol Res The *Journal of Obstetrics and Gynaecology* is an international peer-reviewed medical journal that publishes original research and review articles on the entire field of obstetrics and gynecology, with an emphasis on practical applicability. The journal publishes a wide range of papers, including scientific and clinical research, reviews, case reports, and supplements on clinical symposia.

J Psychiatry Med *The International Journal of Psychiatry in Medicine* bridges the gap between clinical psychiatry research and primary care clinical research. The relevance of psychobiological, psychological, social, familial, religious, and cultural factors in the development and treatment of illness; the relationship of biomarkers to psychiatric symptoms and syndromes in primary care; research on dealing with the challenges of managing psychiatric syndromes in the setting of multiple medical co-morbidities; the impact of financial and technological changes in clinical practice on the broad scope of psychiatry health care; the significance and meaning of disease to the emotional and psychological state of individuals, and medical education research that helps prepare future practitioners to address these issues.

J Psychosom Res The *Journal of Psychosomatic Research* is a multidisciplinary research journal covering all aspects of the relationships between psychology and medicine. The scope is broad and ranges from basic human biological and psychological research to evaluations of treatment and services.

Lancet Psychiatry *The Lancet Psychiatry* publishes original research that advocates change in, or illuminates, psychiatric practice. Topics considered by the journal include psychopharmacology, psychotherapy, and psychosocial approaches to all psychiatric disorders, across the life course. We cover innovative treatments and the biological research underpinning such developments, novel methods of service delivery, and new ways of thinking about mental illness promoted by social psychiatry.

Lancet Public Health *The Lancet Public Health* is committed to tackling the most pressing issues across all aspects of public health. In particular, and in line with the values and vision of *The Lancet*, we have a strong commitment to using science to improve health equity and social justice. We take a broad and inclusive approach to public health, and we are interested in interdisciplinary research. We publish a range of content types including Articles, Review, Comment, and Correspondence that can advance public health policies and outcomes.

Med Care *Medical Care* is a peer-reviewed public health journal that covers the field of health care. It is the official journal of the Medical Care Section of the American Public Health Association.

PLoS One *PLOS One* (stylized *PLOS ONE*, and formerly *PLoS ONE*) is a peer-reviewed open access mega journal published by the Public Library of Science (PLOS) since 2006. The journal covers primary research from any discipline within science and medicine.

Psychiatry Clin Neurosci *Psychiatry and Clinical Neurosciences (PCN)* is a bimonthly peer-reviewed medical journal covering psychiatry and neuroscience.

Psychiatry Res *Psychiatry Research* is a peer-reviewed medical journal covering psychiatry. It was established in 1979 and is published 21 times per year by Elsevier. A section of the journal, *Psychiatry Research: Neuroimaging*, covers the discipline of neuroimaging as it pertains to psychiatry.

Psychiatr Serv *Psychiatric Services* is a monthly peer-reviewed medical journal covering research on psychiatry. It is published by the American Psychiatric Association.

Psychooncology The *Journal of Psychosocial Oncology* is an essential source for up-to-date clinical and research material geared toward health professionals who provide psychosocial services to cancer patients, their families, and their caregivers.

Psychother Psychosom Psychotherapy and Psychosomatics is a bimonthly peer-reviewed medical journal covering psychotherapy and psychosomatic medicine.

R. Curr Psychiatry Rep *Current Psychiatry Reports* is a bimonthly peer-reviewed medical journal publishing review articles related to psychiatry.

Scand J Gastroenterol The Scandinavian Journal of Gastroenterology is a monthly peer-reviewed medical journal covering the field of gastroenterology.

Schizophr Res Schizophrenia Research is a peer-reviewed medical journal covering research on the cause, clinical diagnostics, and treatment of schizophrenia. It is an official journal of the Schizophrenia International Research Society.

Soc Sci Med Social Science & Medicine is a peer-reviewed academic journal covering social science research on health, including anthropology, economics, geography, psychology, social epidemiology, social policy, sociology, medicine and health care practice, policy, and organization.

Soc Psychiatry Psychiatr Epidemiol Social Psychiatry and Psychiatric Epidemiology is a monthly peer-reviewed medical journal covering the epidemiology of psychiatric disorders. It was established in 1966 under the name Social Psychiatry, obtaining its current name in 1988.

Support Care Cancer Supportive Care in Cancer is a monthly peer-reviewed medical journal covering research on cancer care.

Urol Oncol The *Journal of Urologic Oncology* (JUO) publishes practical, timely, and relevant clinical and basic science research articles addressing any aspect of urologic oncology. JUO is of interest to urologists, oncologists, radiologists, and clinicians treating patients and to those involved in research on diseases of urologic oncology. JUO publishes original articles, review articles, editorials, rapid communications, brief reports, and letters.

C. AUTHORS AND INSTITUTIONAL AFFILIATIONS

(800+ internationally published oncologists and cognate scientists) This list constitutes a major roster of published research scholars. *Because each one of these research scholars has been referenced in this book, it seems appropriate to identify each one and the relevant institutional attachment during which time the research was published.*

Abdelaziz, S. Huntsman Cancer Institute, University of Utah School of Medicine, UT

Abuelo, Carolina Internal Medicine, Harvard Medical School, Boston, MA

Ackerman, M.G. Langone Medical Center, New York University, NY

Acruso, Rosangela Institute of Psychiatry, University of Ferrara (Italy)

Adami, H.O. Medical Epidemiology & Biostatistics, Karolinska Institutet, Stockholm (Sweden)

Aguilar-Gaxiola, S. School of Psychology, Interdisciplinary Center IDC), Herzliya (Israel)

Ahlgren-Rimpilainen, A.J. National Institute for Health, Helsinki (Finland)

Ahmedani, B.K. Center for Health Policy Research, Henry Ford Health, Detroit, MI

Akinyemi, E.O. Dept. of Psychiatry, Henry Ford Health, Detroit, MI

Al-Hamzawi, A.O. Bamford Centre for Mental Health, University of Ulster, Londonderry

Alici, Yesne Psychiatry & Behavioral Sciences, Sloan Kettering Cancer Center, NY

Alonso, J. Bamford Centre for Mental Health, University of Ulster, Londonderry (UK)

Alotiby, M. K. N. School of Public Health, University of Queensland, Brisbane (Australia)

Al-Qurayshi, Z. Head & Neck Surgery, University of Iowa Hospitals, Iowa City, IA

Andersson, T.M.L. Medical Epidemiology, Karolinska Institutet, Stockholm (Sweden)

Andreassen, P. Danis National Center for Obesity, Aarhus (Denmark)

Andrade, L.H. School of Psychology, Interdisciplinary Center IDC), Herzliya (Israel)

Arendt, L.H. Public Health,Epidemiology, Aarhus University, Aarhus (Denmark)

Arffman, M. National Institute for Health, Helsinki (Finland)

Arigami, T. Kagoshima University School of Medical Sciences, Kagoshima (Japan)

Angermeyer, M.C. School of Psychology, Interdisciplinary Center IDC), Herzliya (Israel)

Arnautovska, U. School of Clinical Medicine, University of Queensland, Brisbane (Australia)

Ashburner, Jeffrey M. Internal Medicine, Harvard Medical School, Boston, MA

Ashmore, Russell College of Health, Sheffield Hallam University, Sheffield (UK)

Ashworth, Mark Public Health Sciences, King's College London (UK)

Atlas, Steven J. Internal Medicine, Harvard Medical School, Boston, MA

Austin, Coe Columbia University Medical Center, NY

Avila, J.C. Preventive Medicine, University of Texas Medical Branch, Galveston, TX

Ba, Djibril Public Health Sciences, College of Medicine, Penn. State University, Hershey, PA

Bailly, Gregory Dept. of Urology, Dalhousie University, Halifax, NS (Canada)

Baraghoshi, D. Huntsman Cancer Institute, University of Utah School of Medicine, UT

Barley, Elizabeth Nursing & Midwifery, King's College London (UK)

Barry, Maura J. University of New England College of Osteopathic Medicine, ME

Bayon, Rodrigo Head & Neck Surgery, University of Iowa Hospitals, Iowa City, IA

Beck, A.L. Institute for Health Research, Kaiser Permanente Colorado, Aurora, CO

Bekele, S.B. Oncology, Addis Ababa University College of Health Sciences, Addis Ababa

Bell, David Dept. of Urology, Dalhousie University, Halifax, NS (Canada)

Bentson, T.M. Central Denmark Region, Aahus (Denmark)

Berardi, D. Biomedical & Neuromotor Scs., University of Bologna (Italy)

Bernkley, Tomm Institute of Clinical Medicine, University of Oslo (Norway)

Berstad, Paula Cancer Registry of Norway, Oslo (Norway)

Bertelli, Tatiana Intituto Scientifico Romagnolo per lo Studio, Meldola (Italy)

Bhandarkar, Archis. Alix School of Medicine, May Clinic, Scottsdale, AZ

Bhattacharya, M. Healthcare Delivery Research, National Cancer Institute, Rockville, MD

Biancosino, Bruno S. Anna University Hospital and Local Health Trust, Ferrara (Italy)

Blaes, Anne Hematology/Oncology, University of MN Medical School, Minneapolis, MN

Blaschke, K. Faculty of Medicine & University Hospital, University of Cologne (GER)

Bobo, William V. Psychiatry and Psychology, Mayo Clinic, Jacksonville, FL

Boehncke, A. Medical Psychology, University Medical Center, Leipzig (GER)

Bokemeyer, C. Oncology, University Medical Center, Hamburg (Germany)

Bogner, Emma Sunnybrook Research Institute, Toronto, Ontario (Canada)

Bondergaard, K.B. Central Denmark Region, Aahus (Denmark)

Borges, T.L. College of Nursing, University of Sao Paulo (BRAZIL)

Bortolotti, Lisa Dept. of Philosophy, Institute of Mental Health, University of Birmingham (UK)

Boscoe, F.P. Biostatistics, School of Public Health, State University of New York, NY

Botteri, Edoardo Cancer Registry of Norway, Oslo (Norway)

Bowes, David Radiation Oncology, Dalhousie University, Halifax, NS (Canada)

Brahler, E. Medical Psychology, University Medical Center, Leipzig (GER)

Broadbent, M.T.M. King's College London (Institute of Psychiatry), London, UK
Brogaard, T. Gellerup Medical Practice, Aarhus (Denmark)
Brophy, Lisa Allied Health, Human Services/Sport, La Trobe University, Melbourne (Australia)
Bruffaerts, R. Bamford Centre for Mental Health, University of Ulster, Londonderry (UK)
Bruun, J.M. Dept. of Oncology, Aarhus University Hospital, Aarhus (Denmark)
Buigues, C. Dept. of Nursing, Faculty of Nursing & Chiropody, University of Valencia (Spain)
Busby, John Public Health, Royal Victoria Hospital, Belfast (No. Ireland)
Bydon, Mohamad Dept. of Neurologic Surgery, Mayo Clinic, Rochester, MN
Cabassa, L. J. Columbia School of Social Work (NY)
Call, Kathleen University of Minnesota School of Public Health, Minneapolis, MN
Callaway, Catherine A. Psychiatry, Massachusetts General Hospital, Boston, MA
Cardwell, C.R. Public Health, Royal Victoria Hospital, Belfast (No. Ireland)
Carnahan, R.M. Epidemiology, College of Public Health, University of Iowa, IA
Caruso, Rosangela Institute of Psychiatry, University of Ferrara (Italy)
Carvalho, A.F. Dept. of Psychiatry, University of Toronto, ONT (Canada)
Cauli, O. Dept. of Nursing, Faculty of Nursing & Chiropody, University of Valencia (Spain)
Cespedes, P. Dept. of Nursing, Faculty of Nursing & Chiropody, University of Valencia (Spain)

Chang, Chun-Pin Huntsman Cancer Institute, Salt Lake City, UT

Chang, C-K. King's College London (Institute of Psychiatry), London, UK

Charlesworth, Laura College of Health, Sheffield Hallam University, Sheffield (UK)

Chochinov, Harvey M. Psychiatry, University of Manitoba, Winnipeg, Manitoba (Canada)

Chou, F.H-C. Community Psychiatry, Kaohsiung Municipal Psychiatric Hospital (Taiwan)

Chrischilles, E.A. Epidemiology, College of Public Health, University of Iowa, IA

Chung, W-S. Health Services Admin., China Medical University, Taichung (Taiwan)

Cloyd, Jordan M. Surgical Oncology, Wesner Medical Center, Ohio State University (USA)

Coburn, Natalie G. Dept. of Surgery, University of Toronto, Ontario (Canada)

Collings, Sunny Social Psychiatry & Mental Health Research, University of Otago (NZ)

Consedine, Nathan S. Psychological Medicine, University of Auckland (NZ)

Conwell, Y. Dept. of Psychiatry, University of Rochester School of Medicine, NY

Coomarasamy, Christin Ko Awatea, Counties Manukau Health, Auckland (NZ)

Corona, Patricia Harvard Medical School, Boston, MA

Correll, C.U. Dept. of Psychiatry, Zucker Hillside Hospital, Glen Oaks, NY (US)

Corveleyn, Amy E. Psychiatry, Massachusetts General Hospital, Boston, MA

Crew, Katherine D. Columbia University Medical Center, NY

Cui, Yongjia Oncology, Academy of Chinese Medical Scs., Guang'anmen Hospital (China)

Cummings, J.R. Emory University Rollins School of Public Health, Atlanta, GA

Cunningham, Amy T. Community Medicine, Thomas Jefferson Univer., Philadelphia (USA)

Cunningham, Ruth Public Health, University of Otago ,Wellington (NZ)

Czene, Kamila Medical Epidemiology, Karolinska Institutet, Stockholm (Sweden)

Daida, Y.G. Center for Health Research, Kaiser Permanente Hawaii, Honolulu, HI

D'Alton, P. School of Psychology, University College Dublin (Ireland)

Dalton, S. O. Danish Cancer Society Research Center, Kobenhavn (Denmark)

Danker, H. Psychosocial Oncology, University Medical Center, Leipzig (Germany)

Daumit, Gail Psychiatry & Behavioral Scs., Johns Hopkins School of Medicine (USA)

Davies, E. King's College London (Institute of Psychiatry), London, UK

Davis, Laura E. Sunnybrook Research Institute, Toronto, Ontario (Canada)

De Girolamo, G Bamford Centre for Mental Health, University of Ulster, Londonderry (UK)

De Jonge, P. Bamford Centre for Mental Health, University of Ulster, Londonderry (UK)

De Lange, Thomas Dept. of Medical Reserch, Baerum Hospital, Gjettum (Norway)

Demissie, K. Epidemiology, Rutgers School of Public Health, Piscataway, NJ

De Padova, Silvia Intituto Scientifico Romagnolo per lo Studio, Meldola (Italy)

De Oliveira, J.I. Prefeitura Municipal de Barretos, Municippal de Saude, Sao Paulo (BRAZIL)

De Oliveira, P.A. Prefeitura Municipal de Barretos, Municippal de Saude, Sao Paulo (BRAZIL)

De Rossi, F. Biomedical & Neuromotor Scs., University of Bologna (Italy)

Deshmukh, V. University of Utah Health Care CMIO Office, UT

Deshpande, A.J. Alix School of Medicine, May Clinic, Scottsdale, AZ

Diaz, A. Surgery, Wesner Medical Center, Ohio State University, Columbus, OH

Dietz, A. Otorhinolaryngology/HNS, University Medical Center, Leipzig (Germany)

Dillhoff, Mary E. Surgical Oncology, Wesner Medical Center, Ohio State University (USA)

Donnelly, A. School of Psychology, University College Dublin (Ireland)

Donnelly, M.J.C. Centre for Public Health, Queen's University Belfast (UK)

Dos Santos, J.C. Santa Casa de Misericordia, Barretos, Sao Paulo (BRAZIL)

Dragioti, E. Medicine & Health Scs., Linkoping University (Sweden)

Dresen, Antje Faculty of Medicine, Medical Sociology, University of Cologne (GER)

Du, Zhicheng Biostatistics, School of Public Health, State University of New York, NY

Ejaz, Aslam Surgical Oncology, Wesner Medical Center, Ohio State University (USA)

El-Gabalawy, R. Psychology, Faculty of Arts, University of Manitoba (Canada)

Endeshaw, M. Program of Public Health, Rift Valley University, Addis Ababa (Ethiopia)

Erichsen, Rune Dept. of Surgery, Randers Regional Hospital (Denmark)

Ernst, Andreas Dept. of Epidemiology, University of California, Los Angeles, CA

Etoh, T. Dept. of Nursing, Shimane University Hospital, Izumo (Japan)

Euler, S. Psychiatry & Psychosomatic Medicine, University Hospital Zurich (Switzerland)

Fall, K. Medical Epidemiology & Biostatistics, Karolinska Institutet, Stockholm (Sweden)

Faller, H. Medical Psychology, University Medical Center, Leipzig (GER)

Fan, Yunhua Dept. of Urology, University of Minnesota, MN

Fang, F. Medical Epidemiology & Biostatistics, Karolinska Institutet, Stockholm (Sweden)

Fegan, Colette College of Health, Sheffield Hallam University, Sheffield (UK)

Felton, J.W. Center for Health Policy Research, Henry Ford Health, Detroit, MI

Ferrara, Maria S. Anna University Hospital and Local Health Trust, Ferrara (Italy)

Feyera, F. Psychiatry, Ambo University College of Medicine and Health Science (Ethiopia)

Fiedorowicz, J.G. Epidemiology, College of Public Health, University of Iowa, IA

Fields, Lauren E. Psychiatry, Massachusetts General Hospital, Boston, MA

Fioritti, A. Dept. of Mental Health, Local Health Trust of Bologna (Italy)

Firth, Joseph Health Research, Western Sydney University, NSW (Australia)

Floe, L.E. Dept. of Oncology, Aarhus University Hospital, Aarhus (Denmark)

Flores, E.J. Radiology, Massachusetts General Hospital/Harvard Medical School, Boston, MA

Florescu, S. School of Psychology, Interdisciplinary Center IDC), Herzliya (Israel)

Folesani, Federica Institute of Psychiatry, University of Ferrara (Italy)

Fornaro, Michele Young Mental Health, University of Melbourne, VIC (Australia)

Frank, C.B. Dept. of Psychiatry, Henry Ford Health, Detroit, MI

Fraser, A.M. Population Science, Huntsman Cancer Institute, UT School of Medicine, UT

Fried, D.A. Epidemiology, State University of New Jersey, Newark, NJ

Frison, E. Medicine & Surgery, University of Padua (Italy)

Frolov, L. Dept. of Psychiatry, Weill Institute, University of California, San Francisco, CA

Fujimori, M. National Cancer Center Institute for Cancer Control, Tokyo (Japan)

Fujiwara, M. Dept. of Neuropsychiatry, Okayama University School of Medicine (Japan)

Fuller-Thomson, E. Faculty of Social Work, University of Toronto (Canada)

Fuscar-Poli, P. Institute of Psychiatry, King's College London (UK)

Gaffney, David Population Sciences, University of UT School of Medicine, Salt Lake City, UT

Galway, K. School of Nursing and Midwifery, QUB (UK)

Garrido-Languna, I. Dept. of Internal Medicine, Univ. of Utah School of Medicine, UT

Gilcrease, G.W. Dept. of Internal Medicine, Univ. of Utah School of Medicine, UT

Gennimata, V. Dept. of Microbiology, School of Medicine, University of Athens (Greece)

Geue, K. Medical Psychology & Sociology, University Medical Center, Leipzig (Germany)

Gillis, Charles Dept. of Urology, Dalhousie University, Halifax, NS (Canada)

Gissler, Mika Neurobiology, Family Medicine, Karolinska Institute, Stockholm (Sweden)

Giordano, S.H. MD Andersen Cancer Center, University of Texas, Houston, TX

Glaesmer, H. Medical Psychology, University Medical Center, Leipzig (Germany)

Grassi, Luigi Institute of Psychiatry, Biomedical Sciences, University of Ferrara (Italy)

Green, C.A. Northwest Center for Health Research, Portland, OR

Greer, Joseph A. Harvard Medical School, Boston, MA

Gregorio, Sharla Internal Medicine, Wexner Medical Center, Ohio State University (USA)

Groome, Pattie A. Public Health Sciences, Queen's University, Kingston, Ontario (Canada)

Gu, Dian MD Andersen Cancer Center, University of Texas, Houston, TX

Gunther, M.P. Psychiatry & Psychosomatic Medicine, University Hospital Zurich (Switzerland)

Guntinas-Lichius, O. Otorhinolaryngology/HNS, University Hospital, Jena (Germany)

Guo, Liping School of Basic Medical Sciences, Lanzhou University (China)

Gupta, Ayushi Kasturba Medical College, Mangalore (India)

Gupta, Sumit Hospital for Sick Children, Toronto (Canada)

Gureje, Oye School of Psychology, Interdisciplinary Center IDC), Herzliya (Israel)

Hammelef, K. Institute of Psychiatry, Specialty Surgical Sciences, University of Ferrara (Italy)

Han, Xuesong Health Services Research, American Cancer Society, Atlanta, GA

Hanna, Timothy P. Dept. of Oncology, Queen's University, Kingston, Ontario (Canada)

Hanson, G.C. Johns Hopkins University, Baltimore, MD

Harter, M. Medical Psychology, University Medical Center, Leipzig (GER)

Hashibe, Mia Huntsman Cancer Institute, University of Utah School of Medicine, UT

Haskins, C.B. Epidemiology, College of Public Health, University of Iowa, IA

Hayes, Joseph F. Dept. of Psychiatry, University College London (UK)

Hayes, R.D. King's College London (Institute of Psychiatry), London, UK

He, Weiguo MD Andersen Cancer Center, University of Texas, Houston, TX

He, Yanling School of Psychology, Interdisciplinary Center IDC), Herzliya (Israel)

Helmer, D. NJ Medical School, State University of New Jersey, Newark, NJ

Hemington, Amy Psychology & Social Work, Counties Manukau Health, Auckland (NZ)

Henderson, Max J. Psychiatry, King's College London (UK)

Herweijer, Eva Environmental Medicine, Karolinska Institutet, Stockholm (Sweden)

Hicks, B.M. Public Health, Royal Victoria Hospital, Belfast (No. Ireland)

Higuchi, Y. Taiyo Hills Hospital, Takahashi (Japan)

Hinotsu, S. Biostatistics/Data Management, Sapporo Medical University, Sapporo (Japan)

Hirata, M. Kagoshima University School of Medical Sciences, Kagoshima (Japan)

Hirshfield, K.M. Rutgers Cancer Institute of New Jersey, New Brunswick, NJ

Hoff, Geir Institute of Clinical Medicine, University of Oslo (Norway)

Holme, Oyyind Dept. of Medicine, Sorlandet Hospital, Hristiansand (Norway)

Horii, S. Zikei Hospital, Okayama (Japan)

Hosler, A. S. Biostatistics, School of Public Health, State University of New York, NY

Hotopf, M. King's College London (Institute of Psychiatry), London, UK

Hu, Chivi Bamford Centre for Mental Health, University of Ulster, Londonderry (UK)

Hu, Kejia Environmental Medicine, Karolinska Institutet, Stockholm (Sweden)

Hu, Siqi Huntsman Cancer Institute, Salt Lake City, UT

Huang, Daisy Psychological Medicine, University of Auckland (NZ)

Huang, L.C. Dept. of Surgery, Huntsman Cancer Institute, University of Utah, UT

Hultman, C.M. Medical Epidemiology, Karolinska Institutet, Stockholm (Sweden)

Hund, B. Medical Psychology, University Medical Center, Leipzig (GER)

Huovinen, R. Oncology & Radiotherapy, Turku University Hospital, Turku (Finland)

Hurley, Katelyn E. Community Medicine, Thomas Jefferson University, Philadelphia (USA)

Hyer, J. Madison Surgical Oncology, Wesner Medical Center, Ohio State University (USA)

Idos, Gregory Gastroenterology & Hepatology, Keck School of Medicine, USC, CA

Iglay, Kristy Epidemiology, Rutgers School of Public Health, Piscataway, NJ

Ihle, Peter Faculty of Medicine & University Hospital, University of Cologne (GER)

Ikeda, Y. Obstetrics/Gyn., Nagoya University School of Medicine, Nagoya (Japan)

Ilie, Gabriella Health and Epidemiology, Dalhousie University, Halifax, NS (Canada)

Inagaki, M. Psychiatry, Faculty of Medicine, Shimane University, Izumo (Japan)

Inoue, S. Dept. of Neuropsychiatry, Okayama University School of Medicine (Japan)

Irwin, Kelly E. Psychiatry, Massachusetts General Hospital, Boston, MA

Jacobs, Jamie M. Harvard Medical School, Boston, MA

James, M. Dept. of Psychiatry, Weill Institute, University of California, San Francisco, CA

Jarosek, Stephanie L. Dept. of Urology, University of Minnesota, MN

Jellestad, L. Psychiatry & Psychosomatic Medicine, University Hospital Zurich (Switzerland)

Ji, Xu Pediatrics, Emory University School of Medicine, Atlanta, GA

Johnsen, S.P. Clinical Medicine, Aalborg University & Hosppital, Aalborg (Denmark)

Jones, Alex Dept. of Health and Social Care, London (UK)

Jones, M.P. Royal Hobart Hospital, Hobart (Australia)

Jordan, S. J. QIMR Berghofer Medical Research Institute, Brisbane (Australia)

Jorgensen, Marie D. Clinical Epidemiology, Aarhus University Hospital (Denmark)

Kahn, G.D. Center for Health Policy Research, Henry Ford Health, Detroit, MI

Kajiyama, H. Obstetrics/Gyn., Nagoya University School of Medicine, Nagoya (Japan)

Kakeda, K. Neuropsychiatry, Kochi Medical School, Kochi University, Nankoku (Japan)

Kandil, Emad Surgery, Tulane University School of Medicine, New Orleans, LA

Karam, E.G. School of Psychology, Interdisciplinary Center IDC), Herzliya (Israel)

Kaster, T.S. Psychiatry, Faculty of Medicine, University of Toronto (Canada)

Kaul, Sapna Preventive Medicine, University of Texas Medical Branch, Galveston, TX

Kebede, Y. University of Gondar College of Medicine and Health Science, Gondar (Ethiopia)

Keller, M. Medical Psychology, University Medical Center, Leipzig (GER)

Kelly, E.P. Surgery, Wesner Medical Center, Ohio State University, Columbus, OH

Kendall, B. J. Gastroenterology & Hepatology, Princess Alexandra Hospital, Brisbane (AUS)

Kennedy-Hendricks, Alene Health Policy, Johns Hopkins Bloomberg School, Baltimore, MD

Kerrison, R.S. School of Health Scs., University of Surrey, Guildford, Surrey (UK)

Keskimaki, I. National Institute, Health & Social Systems Research, Helsinki (Finland)

Kessler, R.C. Bamford Centre for Mental Health, University of Ulster, Londonderry (UK)

Keszte, J. Psychosocial Oncology, University Medical Center, Leipzig (Germany)

Kiejna, A. Bamford Centre for Mental Health, University of Ulster, Londonderry (UK)

Kijima, Y. Kagoshima University School of Medical Sciences, Kagoshima (Japan)

Kikkawa, F. Obstetrics/Gyn., Nagoya University School of Medicine, Nagoya (Japan)

Kim, H. Laboratory Medicine, Pusan National University Hospital, Busan (ROK)

Kim, Y. H. Laboratory Medicine, Pusan National University Hospital, Busan (ROK)

Kirchhoff, A.C. Research, Huntsman Cancer Institute, University of Utah, Salt Lake City, UT

Kirkoen, Benedicte Cancer Registry of Norway, Oslo (Norway)

Kisely, Steve School of Clinical Medicine, University of Queensland, Brisbane (Australia)

Kisely, S. Psychiatry, Community Health, Dalhousie University, Halifax (Canada)

Keskimaki, I. Faculty of Social Sciences, Tampere University, Tampere (Finland)

Kittel, Julie A. Health Sciences, University of Rochester School of Medicine, NY

Knudsen, Amy Technology Assessment, Harvard Medical School, Boston, MA

Koivunen, J. National Institute, Health & Social Systems Research, Helsinki (Finland)

Koch, U. Medical Psychology, University Medical Center, Leipzig (GER)

Koczwara, B. Medical Oncology, Flinders Medical Centre,Adelaide (AUS)

Kodama, M. Okayama Psychiatric Medical Center, Okayama (Japan)

Konety, Isha Dept. of Urology, University of Minnesota, MN

Kovanagi, A. Parc Sanitari Sant Joan de Deu, Universitat de Barcelona (Spain)

Kuhnt, S. Medical Psychology, University Medical Center, Leipzig (GER)

Kulharni, V. Community Medicine, Kasturba Medical College, Mangalore (India)

Kuliszewski, M.G. School of Public Health, State University of New York, NY

Kunheri, Beena NCCCR Hamad Medical Corporation, Doha (Qatar)

Kunheri, Beena Medical Oncology, Amrita Institute of Medical Sciences, Kochi (India)

Kurahara, H. Kagoshima University School of Medical Sciences, Kagoshima (Japan)

Kurdyak, Paul Depart. Of Psychhiatry, University of Toronto, Toronto, Ontario (Canada)

Larsen, J. T. Ntl. Centre for Register-Based Research, Aarhus University (Denmark)

Lau, Cindy ICES, Toronto (Canada)

Launders, Naomi Dept. of Psychiatry, University College London (UK)

Laursen, T. M. Ntl. Centre for Register-Based Research, Aarhus University (Denmark)

Lawen, Joseph Dept. of Urology, Dalhousie University, Halifax, NS (Canada)

Lawrence, D. Graduate School of Education, University of Western Australia, Perth (Australia)

Lawrence, W.R. School of Public Health, State University of New York, NY

Leahy, D. School of Psychology, University College Dublin (Ireland)

Lee, J.H. Medical Student, College of Medicine, Penn. State University, Hershey, PA

Leinung, M.C. Dept. of Medicine, Medical College, Albany, NY

Lepine, J-P., Bamford Centre for Mental Health, University of Ulster, Londonderry (UK)

Lera-Calatayud, G. Nursing, Faculty of Nursing & Chiropody, University of Valencia (Spain)

Leslie, Douglas Public Health Scs, College of Medicine, Penn. State University, Hershey, PA

Levav, Itzhak School of Psychology, Interdisciplinary Center IDC), Herzliya (Israel)

Levinson, D. Bamford Centre for Mental Health, University of Ulster, Londonderry (UK)

Liberante, F.G. Centre for Cancer Research, Queen's University Belfast (No. Ireland)

Li, Jiong Clinical Epidemiology, Aarhus University & Hospital (Denmark)

Li, Meixuan School of Basic Medical Sciences, Lanzhou University (China)

Li, Yanfei School of Basic Medical Sciences, Lanzhou University (China)

Li, Zhihong School of Basic Medical Sciences, Lanzhou University (China)

Lim, Carmen Bamford Centre for Mental Health, University of Ulster, Londonderry (UK)

Lin, Yong Biostatistics, Rutgers School of Public Health, Piscataway, NJ

Liu, Guodong Public Health Scs, College of Medicine, Penn. State University, Hershey, PA

Logan, H. School of Clinical Medicine, University of Queensland, Brisbane (Australia)

Lloyd, Shane Radiation Oncology, University of Utah School of Medicine, UT

Lu, C.Y. Population Medicine, Harvard Medical School, Health Care Institute, Boston, MA

Lu, Donghao Medical Epidemiology, Karolinska Institutet, Stockholm (Sweden)

Lu, Wenping Oncology, Academy of Chinese Medical Scs., Guang'anmen Hospital (China)

Lugton, Cam Dept. of Health and Social Care, London (UK)

Lumme, S. National Institute for Health, Helsinki (Finland)

Lustberg, Maryam Surgical Oncology, Wesner Medical Center, Ohio State University (USA)

Lynch, F.L. Center for Health Research, Kaiser Permanente Hawaii, Portland, OR

Ma, K-J. Dept. of Public Health, China Medical University, Taichung (Taiwan)

Maemura, K. Kagoshima University School of Medical Sciences, Kagoshima (Japan)

Magnuson, A. Dept. of Medicine, University of Rochester School of Medicine, NY

Maguire, Aideen Centre for Public Health, Queen's University Belfast (UK)

Mahar, Alyson L. Health Scs., University of Manitoba College of Medicine (Canada)

Mairs, Adrian Public Health Agency Northern Ireland, Belfast (UK)

Malila, Nea Finish Cancer Registry, Helsinki (Finland)

Manderbacka, K. National Institute for Health, Helsinki (Finland)

Mangurian, C. Dept. of Psychiatry, Weill Institute, University of California, San Francisco, CA

Marchak, J.G. Emory University School of Medicine, Atlanta, GA

Marella, Marco Institute of Psychiatry, University of Ferrara (Italy)

Marzaroli, P. Dept. of Public Health, Local Health Trust of Bologna (Italy)

Mason, Ross Dept. of Urology, Dalhousie University, Halifax, NS (Canada)

Matschinger, H. Bamford Centre for Mental Health, University of Ulster, Londonderry (UK)

Matsushita, T. Zikei Hospital, Okayama (Japan)

McAlpine, D. University of Minnesota School of Public Health, Minneapolis, MN

McDowell, B.D. Holden Cancer Center, University of Iowa, Iowa City, IA

McFarland, D.C. Medicine, Northwell Health Cancer Institute, Lenox Hill Hospital, NY

McGinty, Emma A. Mental Health, Johns Hopkins School of Medicine (USA)
McIntosh, S.A. Centre for Cancer Research, Queen's University Belfast (No. Ireland)
McLaughlin, Sarah Dept. of Surgery, Mayo Clinic, Jacksonville, FL
Medina-Mora, M.E. Bamford Centre for Mental Health, University of Ulster, Londonderry
Mehnert, A. Medical Psychology, University Medical Center, Leipzig (GER)
Mehnert-Theuerkauf, A. Medical Psych., University Medical Center, Leipzig (Germany)
Meister, E. Otorhinolaryngology, Clinical Center Sankt Georg, Leipzig (Germany)
Menchetti, M. Biomedical & Neuromotor Scs., University of Bologna (Italy)
Mertens, A.C. Epidemiology, Emory University Rollins School of Public Health, GA
Meyere, A. Psychosocial Oncology, University Medical Center, Leipzig (Germany)
Miasso, A.I. College of Nursing, University of Sao Paulo (BRAZIL)
Mikkelsen, Ellen M. Clinical Epidemiology, Aarhus University Hospital (Denmark)
Millman, J. School of Nursing and Midwifery, QUB (UK)
Mills, Ken Centre for Cancer Research, Queen's University Belfast (No. Ireland)
Mimaki, Y. Dept. of Nursing, Okayama University Hospital, Okayama (Japan)
Mitchell, A.J. Cancer & Molecular Medicine, University of Leicester (UK)

Miola, Alessandro Neurosciences Dept., University of Padua (Italy)

Moller, H. King's College London (Institute of Psychiatry), London, UK

Momen, N.C. Clinical Epidemiology, Aarhus University Hospital, Aarhus (Denmark)

Moriyama, Y. Obstetrics/Gyn., Nagoya University School of Medicine, Nagoya (Japan)

Morgan, J. H. Foundation House/Oxford (UK)

Moskalewicz, J. School of Psychology, Interdisciplinary Center IDC), Herzliya (Israel)

Mota, N. Health Psychology, Faculty of Health Sciences, University of Manitoba (Canada)

Mugadza, V. Cancer & Molecular Medicine, University of Leicester (UK)

Mulligan, C. Psychiatry, Massachusetts General Hospital, Boston, MA

Munk-Olsen, T. Ntl. Centre for Register-Based Research, Aarhus University (Denmark)

Murphy, Karly A. Internal Medicine, Johns Hopkins School of Medicine (USA)

Murphy, Sam School of Psychology, Interdisciplinary Center IDC), Herzliya (Israel)

Murri, Martino B. Institute of Psychiatry, University of Ferrara (Italy)

Musti, M.A. Dept. of Public Health, Local Health Trust of Bologna (Italy)

Mutambudzi, M. Preventive Medicine, University of Texas Medical Branch, Galveston, TX

Muzikansky, A. Biostatistics Center, Mass. General Hospital, Boston, MA

Mygind, A. Research Unit for General Practice, Aarhus (Denmark)

Mystakidou, K. Radiology, Areteion Hospital, School of Medicine, Univ. of Athens (Greece)

Nagoshi, K. Faculty of Medicine, Shimane University, Izumo (Japan)

Nahash, O. School of Psychology, Interdisciplinary Center IDC), Herzliya (Israel)

Nakajo, A. Kagoshima University School of Medical Sciences, Kagoshima (Japan)

Nakamura, Y. School of Psychology, Interdisciplinary Center IDC), Herzliya (Israel)

Nakava, N. Health Sciences, Saitama Prefectural University, Koshigaya (Japan)

Nanni, Mara Giulia Institute of Psychiatry, University of Ferrara (Italy)

Nathan, Paul C. Institute of Health Policy, University of Toronto (Canada)

Natsugoe, S. Kagoshima University School of Medical Sciences, Kagoshima (Japan)

Neergaard, M.A. Palliative Care Unit, Aahus University Hospital, Aarhus (Denmark)

Neil, J. M. Mongan Institute, Massachusetts General Hospital, Boston, MA

Nelson, Zoe E. Psychological Sciences, University of Connecticut, Storrs, CT

Newcomer, J.W. Psychiatry, Weill Institute, University of California, San Francisco, CA

Newman, Michael University of Utah Health Care CMIO Office, UT

Ng, H.S. Medical Research Institute, College of Medicine, Flinders University, Adelaide (AUS)

Niazi, Shehzad Psychiatry and Psychology, Mayo Clinic, Jacksonville, FL

Nie, D. Health Services Admin., China Medical University, Taichung (Taiwan)

Nierenberg, Andrew A. Psychiatry, Massachusetts General Hospital, Boston, MA

Niimi, K. Obstetrics/Gyn., Nagoya University School of Medicine, Nagoya (Japan)

Nishino, K. Obstetrics/Gyn., Nagoya University School of Medicine, Nagoya (Japan)

Nordentoft, M. Lundbeck Foundation for Psychiatric Research, Aarhus (Denmark)

Oechsle, K. Oncology, Palliative Care, University Medical Center, Hamburg (Germany)

Oeken, J. Dept. of Otorhinolaryngology, Clinical Center Chemnitz (Germany)

Olsen, Jorn Clinical Epidemiology, Aarhus University & Hospital (Denmark)

O'Neil, F.A. Public Health, Royal Victoria Hospital, Belfast (No. Ireland)

O'Neill, S. Bamford Centre for Mental Health, University of Ulster, Londonderry (No.IR/UK)

O'Reilly, D.P.J. Centre for Public Health, Queen's University Belfast (UK)

Osborn, David P. J. Dept. of Psychiatry, University College London (UK)

Ostroff, J.S. Psychiatry & Behavioral Scs., Sloan Kettering Cancer Center, NY

Ounalli, Heifa Institute of Psychiatry, University of Ferrara (Italy)

Owen-Smith, A.A. Georgia State University School of Public Health, Atlanta, GA

Pabst, F. Otorhinolaryngology, Dresden-Friedrichstadt, Dresden (Germany)

Pai, Keshva Psychiatry, Kasturba Medical College, Mangalore (India)

Palagini, Laura S. Anna University Hospital and Local Health Trust, Ferrara (Italy)

Palmer, Elizabeth Surgical Oncology, Wesner Medical Center, Ohio State University (USA)

Pandolfi, P. Dept. of Public Health, Local Health Trust of Bologna (Italy)

Pappano, Catherine R. Psychology, University of Colorado, Denver, CO

Paredes, Anghela Z. Surgical Oncology, Wesner Medical Center, Ohio State University (USA)

Park, Elyse R. Mongan Institute for Health Policy, Mass. General Hospital, Boston, MA

Park, Sung Jin Institute of Psychiatry, King's College London (UK)

Parpa, Efi Radiology, School of Medicine, University of Athens (Greece)

Parsons, Helen University of Minnesota School of Public Health, Minneapolis, MN

Patil, Nikhilesh Radiation Oncology, Dalhousie University, Halifax, NS (Canada)

Pavithran, Keechilat Medical Oncology, Amrita Institute of Medical Sciences, Kochi, (India)

Pawlik, Timothy M. Surgical Oncology, The Ohio State University Medical Center (USA)

Pedersen, Lars Clinical Epidemiology, Aarhus University & Hospital (Denmark)

Peng, Jianhe Dept. of Health and Social Care, London (UK)

Pentakota, S.R. Epidemiology, State University of New Jersey, Newark, NJ

Peoples, A.R. Radiation Oncology, University of UT School of Medicine, Salt Lake City, UT

Pepereke, S. Cancer & Molecular Medicine, University of Leicester (UK)

Percac-Lima, Sanja Internal Medicine, Harvard Medical School, Boston, MA

Perez, Giselle K. Mongan Institute for Health Policy, Mass. General Hospital, Boston, MA

Perlangeli, V. Dept. of Public Health, Local Health Trust of Bologna (Italy)

Perrin, N.A. Northwest Center for Health Research, Portland, OR

Peterson, Debbie Social Psychiatry & Mental Health Research, University of Otago (NZ)

Pfaff, Holger Faculty of Medicine, Medical Sociology, University of Cologne (GER)

Pham, Hannah Urology, Texas Tech University Health Scs. Center, Lubbock, TX

Piazza, M. Bamford Centre for Mental Health, University of Ulster, Londonderry (UK)

Pickron, T. B. Dept. of Surgery, Huntsman Cancer Institute, University of Utah, UT

Pirl, William F. Harvard Medical School, Boston, MA

Pole, J.D. Pediatric Oncology Group of Ontario, Toronto (Canada)

Pollack, Craig E. Clinical Research, Johns Hopkins Medical Institutions (USA)

Ponzani, C. Intervention Research Program, Mass. General Hospital, Boston, MA

Posada-Villa, J. Bamford Centre for Mental Health, University of Ulster, Londonderry (UK)
Presskreischer, Rachel Health Policy & Management, Johns Hopkins School of Medicine (US)
Price, Gabriele Dept. of Health and Social Care, London (UK)
Protani, Melinda M. School of Public Health, University of Queensland, Brisbane (Australia)
Pukkala, E. Faculty of Social Sciences, Tampere University, Tampere (Finland)
Ramlau-Hansen, C.H. Public Health,Epidemiology, Aarhus University, Aarhus (Denmark)
Randel, Kristin R. Cancer Registry of Norway, Oslo (Norway)
Rasmussen, A.W. Intervention Research Program, Mass. General Hospital, Boston, MA
Ravindran, A.V. Centre for Addition and Mental Health, Toronto (Canada)
Regan, Susan Harvard Medical School, Boston, MA
Reid, J. School of Nursing and Midwifery, QUB (UK)
Rendon, Ricardo Dept. of Urology, Dalhousie University, Halifax, NS (Canada)
Reuter, K. Medical Psychology, University Medical Center, Leipzig (GER)
Reynolds, Lisa M. Psychological Medicine, University of Auckland (NZ
Rhoads, G.G. Epidemiology, Rutgers School of Public Health, Piscataway, NJ
Riano, N.S. Dept. of Psychiatry, Weill Institute, University of California, San Francisco, CA
Riba, Michelle Dept. of Psychiatry, Psycho-oncology Program, University of Michigan, USA

Richard, M. Medical Psychology, University Medical Center, Leipzig (GER)

Richman, J. Dept. of Psychiatry, University of Rochester School of Medicine, NY

Rigotti, N.A. Harvard Medical School, Boston, MA

Robb, Kathryn A. Institute of Health & Wellbeing, University of Glasgow (UK)

Ross, Emma Centre for Public Health, Queen's University Belfast (UK)

Rossi-Meyer, M. Head & Neck Surgery, University of Iowa Hospitals, Iowa City, IA

Rossom, R.C. Health Partners Institute, Minneapolis, MN

Rowe, Kerry G. Intermountain Healthcare, Salt Lake City, UT

Russell, Heidi Hematology-Oncology, Pediatrics, Baylor College of Medicine, Houston, TX

Rutledge, R.D.H. Radiation Oncology, Dalhousie University, Halifax, NS (Canada)

Ryan, David P. Hematology & Oncology, Mass. General Hospital, Boston, MA

Sabato, Silvana Institute of Psychiatry, University of Ferrara (Italy)

Sadeghi-Nejad, H. VA New Jersey Health Care System, East Orange, NJ

Salm, Sandra Faculty of Medicine, Medical Sociology, University of Cologne (GER)

Samaddeer, N. J. Div. of Gastroenterology & Hepatology, Mayo Clinic, Scottsdale, AZ

Sanchez-Martinez, V. Nursing, Faculty of Nursing & Chiropody, University of Valencia (Spain)

Santorelli, M. L. Epidemiology, Rutgers School of Public Health, Piscataway, NJ

Santo-Pereira, I.E. Cancer & Molecular Medicine, University of Leicester (UK)
Santin, O. School of Nursing and Midwifery, QUB (UK)
Saponaro, A. Health & Social Policies, Emilia-Romagna Region, Bologna (Italy)
Sara, G. Faculty of Medicine and Health, University of Sydney (Australia)
Sareen, J. Psychology, Faculty of Arts, University of Manitoba (Canada)
Sarfati, Diana Dept. of Public Health, University of Otago, Wellington (NZ)
Sathianathen, Niranjan J. Dept. of Urology, University of Minnesota, MN
Saxena, P.U.P. Radiotherapy/Oncology, Kasturba Medical College, Mangalore (India)
Scaife, Courtney Dept. of Surgery, Huntsman Cancer Institute, University of Utah, UT
Schillinger, D. Dept. of Psychiatry, Weill Institute, University of California, San Francisco, CA
Scholten, Nadine Faculty of Medicine, Medical Sociology, University of Cologne (GER)
Schubert, I. Faculty of Medicine & University Hospital, University of Cologne (GER)
Schulz, H. Medical Psychology, University Medical Center, Leipzig (GER)
Schulze, J.B. Psychiatry & Psychosomatic Medicine, University Hospital Zurich (Switzerland)
Schwartz, C.L. Pediatrics, The University of Texas MD Anderson Cancer Center, Houston, TX
Schymura, M.J. Biostatistics, School of Public Health, State University of New York, NY

Scolamiero, Laura Dept. of Psychiatry, University College London (UK)

Scott, K.M. Bamford Centre for Mental Health, University of Ulster, Londonderry (UK)

Sehner, S. Medical Psychology, University Medical Center, Leipzig (GER)

Seplaki, C. L. Health Sciences, University of Rochester School of Medicine, NY

Seth, R. Graduate School of Education, University of Western Australia, Perth (Australia)

Shama, M.A. Surgery, Tulane University School of Medicine, New Orleans, LA

Shao, Tianrui Tianjin University of Traditional Chinese Medicine, Tianjin (China)

Shapiro, P.A. Columbia University Medical Center, NY

Sharma, Pranav Urology, Texas Tech University Health Scs. Center, Lubbock, TX

Shen, Chan MD Andersen Cancer Center, University of Texas, Houston, TX

Shen, S-P. Dept. of Public Health, China Medical University, Taichung (Taiwan)

Shimazu, T. Center for Public Health Sciences, Survivorship Research, Tokyo (Japan)

Shin, J.I. Pediatrics, Yonsei University College of Medicine, Seoul (South Korea)

Shinden, Y. Kagoshima University School of Medical Sciences, Kagoshima (Japan)

Shirama, F.H. College of Nursing, University of Sao Paulo (BRAZIL)

Shiroiski, M. Radiology, Keck Schoolof Medicine, Univ. of So. California, Los Angeles, CA

Shtasel, Derri Division of Psychiatry, Harvard Medical School, Boston, MA

Siantz, E. Family Medicine & Public Health, University of California, San Diego, CA

Silva, T.B. Hospital de Cancer da Fundacao Pio XII, Barretos, Sao Paulo (BRAZIL)

Simon, G.E. Kaiser Permanente Washington Health Research Institute, Seattle, WA

Singer, S. Epidemiology, University Medical Center, Mainz (Germany)

Siskind, Dan School of Clinical Medicine, University of Queensland, Brisbane (Australia)

Sjolander, Arvid Medical Epidemiology, Karolinski Institutet, Stockholm (Sweden)

Smith, B.J. Holden Cancer Center, University of Iowa, Iowa City, IA

Smith, K. R. Population Science, Huntsman Cancer Institute, UT School of Medicine, UT

Snyder, John Intermountain Healthcare, Salt Lake City, UT

Solmi, Marco Neurosciences Dept., University of Padua (Italy)

Sommer, J.L. Psychology, Faculty of Arts, University of Manitoba (Canada)

Soole, Rebecca School of Clinical Medicine, University of Queensland, Brisbane (Australia)

Sorensen, H.T. Clinical Epidemiology, Aarhus University & Hospital (Denmark)

Sparen, Par Medical Epidemiology, Karolinski Institutet, Stockholm (Sweden)

Stanley, James Dept. of Public Health, University of Otago, Wellington (NZ)

Stefancic, Ana Columbia University School of Social Work (NY)

Stein, D.J. School of Psychology, Interdisciplinary Center IDC), Herzliya (Israel)

Stewart, Robert J. Psychiatry, King's College London (UK)

Stivanello, E. Dept. of Public Health, Local Health Trust of Bologna (Italy)

Stone, Elizabeth M. Dept. of Health Policy & Management, Johns Hopkins Medicine (USA)

Streck, J.M. Intervention Research Program, Mass. General Hospital, Boston, MA

Stubbs, B. Cancer & Molecular Medicine, University of Leicester (UK)

Stumbo, S.P. Northwest Center for Health Research, Portland, OR

Su, S-Y. Health Services Admin., China Medical University, Taichung (Taiwan)

Sundstrom, Karin Laboratory Medicine, Karolinska Institutet, Stockholm (Sweden)

Suppli, N. P. Lundbeck Foundation for Psychiatric Research, Aarhus (Denmark)

Sutradhar, Rinku Alla Lana School of Public Health, University of Toronto (Canada)

Suvissari, J. National Institute for Health, Helsinki (Finland)

Suzuki, S. Obstetrics/Gyn., Nagoya University School of Medicine, Nagoya (Japan)

Tabata, M. Respiratory Medicine, Okayama University Hospital, Okayama (Japan)

Tachimori, H. Bamford Centre for Mental Health, University of Ulster, Londonderry (UK)

Taib, M.I. School of Psychology, Interdisciplinary Center IDC), Herzliya (Israel)

Tam, S.H. Dept. of Otolaryngology (HNS), Henry Ford Health, Detroit, MI

Tamauchi, S. Obstetrics/Gyn., Nagoya University School of Medicine, Nagoya (Japan)

Tamura, K. Medical Oncology, Shimane University Hospital, Izumo (Japan)

Tanoue, K. Kagoshima University School of Medical Sciences, Kagoshima (Japan)

Tao, Randa Radiation Oncology, University of Utah School of Medicine, UT

Temel, Jennifer S. Hematology & Oncology, Mass. General Hospital, Boston, MA

Testoni, Ines Applied Psychology, University of Padua (Italy)

Thapar, R. Community Medicine, Kasturba Medical College, Mangalore (India)

Thomas, M. Dept. of Psychiatry, Weill Institute, University of California, San Francisco, CA

Thomsen, Mette K. Clinical Epidemiology, Aarhus University Hospital (Denmark)

Tiberto, Elisa Institute of Psychiatry, University of Ferrara (Italy)

Tiersma, Keena M. University of Washington Medical School, Seattle, WA

Tirfessa, K. Kotebe University of Education, Dept. of Psychology, Addis Ababa (Ethiopia)

Toender, A. Ntl. Centre for Register-Based Research, Aarhus University (Denmark)

Toffanin, Tommaso Institute of Psychiatry, University of Ferrara (Italy)

Torres, Harrison Urology, Texas Tech University Health Scs. Center, Lubbock, TX

Trivedi, M.S. Columbia University Medical Center, NY
Tsai, K-Y. Community Psychiatry, Kaohsiung Municipal Psychiatric Hospital (Taiwan)
Tsilika, Eleni Radiology, School of Medicine, University of Athens (Greece)
Tsilimigras, D. I. Surgical Oncology, Wesner Medical Center, Ohio State University (USA)
Tsung, Allan Surgical Oncology, Wesner Medical Center, Ohio State University (USA)
Tuesley, Jaren M. Health Dept., QIMR Berghofer Medical Research Institute (Australia)
Uchitomi, Y. Psychosocial Care, National Cancer Center Hospital, Tokyo (Japan)
Valdimarsdottir, U. Medical Epidemiology & Biostatistics, Karolinska Institutet, Stockholm
Valsraj, Koravangattu Institute of Psychiatry, King's College London (UK)
Van Alphen, M.U. Psychiatry, Massachusetts General Hospital, Boston, MA
Van Warmerdam, J. Hospital for Sick Children, Toronto (Canada)
Van Wijngaarden, E. Health Sciences, University of Rochester School of Medicine, NY
Vedsted, P. Public Health Research, Aarhus University, Aarhus (Denmark)
Vehling, S. Medical Psychology, University Medical Center, Hamburg (Germany)
Verne, Julia Dept. of Health and Social Care, London (UK)
Vetergaard, M. Public Health, Aarhus University (Denmark)
Videbech, P. Clinical Medicine, University of Copenhagen (Denmark)

Vila-Candel, R. Nursing, Faculty of Nursing & Chiropody, University of Valencia (Spain)
Vinogradov, Sophia Psychiatry, University of Minnesota, MN
Vittinghoff, E. Dept. of Psychiatry, Weill Institute, University of California, San Francisco, CA
Voigt, Louis Critical Care Medicine, Memorial Sloan Kettering Cancer Center, NY
Von Kanel, R. Psychiatry/Psychosomatic Medicine, University Hospital Zurich (Switzerland)
Vora, Hita Preventive Medicine, University of Southern California, Los Angeles, CA
Wada, R. Dept. of Neuropsychiatry, Okayama University School of Medicine (Japan)
Wai, Alisa Institute of Psychiatry, King's College London (UK)
Walker, Z.J. Dept. of Psychiatry, University of Toronto, Toronto (Canada)
Wallace, R.B. Epidemiology, College of Public Health, University of Iowa, IA
Wang, Jiangrong Laboratory Medicine, Karolinska Institutet, Stockholm (Sweden)
Wang, J-Y. Health Services Admin., China Medical University, Taichung (Taiwan)
Wang, Ya'nan Oncology, Academy of Chinese Medical Scs., Guang'anmen Hospital (China)
Waring, Stephen Essentia Institute of Rural Health, Duluth, MN
Wegscheider, S. Medical Psychology, University Medical Center, Leipzig (GER)
Weight, Christopher J. Dept. of Urology, University of Minnesota, MN

Weinstein, Lara Community Medicine, Thomas Jefferson University, Philadelpha (USA)

Weis, J. Medical Psychology, University Medical Center, Leipzig (GER)

Weis, John R. Dept. of Internal Medicine, Univ. of Utah School of Medicine, UT

Wender, R. C. Community Medicine, Thomas Jefferson University, Philadelpha (USA)

West, Jeri J. Faculty of Social Work, University of Toronto (Canada)

Westphal, J. Center for Health Policy Research, Henry Ford Health, Detroit, MI

Whisenant, J. Dept. of Internal Medicine, Univ. of Utah School of Medicine, UT

Wilke, Derek Radiation Oncology, Dalhousie University, Halifax, NS (Canada)

Williams, J.M. Rutgers Robert Wood Johnson Medical School, New Brunswick, NJ

Wittchen, H-U. Medical Psychology, University Medical Center, Leipzig (GER)

Woodhead, Charlotte Psychiatry & Neuroscience, King's College London (UK)

Woodman, R. Medical Research, College of Medicine, Flinders University, Adelaide (AUS)

Wu, Brian Keck School of Medicine, University of Southern California, Los Angeles, CA

Wu, H-C. Community Psychiatry, Kaohsiung Municipal Psychiatric Hospital (Taiwan)

Xue, S. Dept. of Psychiatry, University of Toronto, Toronto (Canada)

Yadegarfar, M. Cancer & Molecular Medicine, University of Leicester (UK)

Yamada, Y. Dept. of Neuropsychiatry, Okayama University School of Medicine (Japan)

Yang, Kehu School of Basic Medical Sciences, Lanzhou University (China)

Yao, C-Y. Attending Physician, Psychiatry, An-non Hospital, Tainan (Taiwan)

Yarborough, B.J.H. Northwest Center for Health Research, Portland, OR

Yoshihara, M. Obstetrics/Gyn., Nagoya University School of Medicine, Nagoya (Japan)

Yoshikawa, N. Obstetrics/Gyn., Nagoya University School of Medicine, Nagoya (Japan)

Yoshimura, Y. Zikei Hospital, Okayama (Japan)

Young, Marie J. Psychology & Social Work, Counties Manukau Health, Auckland (NZ)

Zacharia, B.E. Neurosurgery, College of Medicine, Penn. State University, Hershey, PA

Zarkov, Z. School of Psychology, Interdisciplinary Center IDC), Herzliya (Israel)

Zhang, S-D. Biomedical Sciences Research Institute, University of Ulster, Londonderry (No.IR)

Zhang, Weixuan Oncology, Academy of Chinese Medical Scs., Guang'anmen Hospital (China)

Zhang, X. Cancer Epidemiology, New York State Dept. of Health, Albany, NY

Zhang, W. Biostatistics, School of Public Health, State University of New York, NY

Zhu, J. Medical Epidemiology & Biostatistics, Karolinska Institutet, Stockholm (Sweden)

Zhou, Sh. College of Medicine, Penn State University, Hershey, PA

Zhuo, Zhili Oncology, Academy of Chinese Medical Scs., Guang'anmen Hospital (China)

D. TOP CANCER RESEARCH CENTERS

(Descriptions of the listed institutions constitute an aggregation of information gleaned from institutional websites, Google, and Wikipedia sources and are presented as a brief indication of the scope of the institutions' work.)

MD Anderson Cancer Center at the University of Texas is a comprehensive cancer center in Houston, Texas, and is the largest cancer research and treatment center in the United States. It is one of the original three comprehensive cancer centers in the U.S. and is both a degree-granting academic institution and a cancer treatment and research center located at the Texas Medical Center in Houston. It is presently considered the best hospital in the world for oncology and related cancer treatment according to authoritative sources evaluating world treatment centers.

Memorial Sloan-Kettering Cancer Center is a cancer research and treatment institutions in the city of New York which was founded in 1884 as the New York Cancer Hospital. It is one of 52 National Cancer Institute-designated Comprehensive Cancer Centers and its main campus is located at 1275 York Avenue in Manhattan, NY. According to recognized sources for evaluation such as the U.S. News and World Report, this Cancer Center is ranked as the second-best hospital for cancer care in the United States after MD Anderson Cancer Center.

Dana-Farber Cancer Institute is a comprehensive cancer research and treatment institution in Boston, Massachusetts, an affiliate of Harvard University's Comprehensive Cancer Center as designated by the National Cancer Institute and constitutes one of the 15 clinical affiliates and research institutes of Harvard Medical School. By the leading ranking agencies, it holds the 4th position as a cancer hospital in the world boasting an internationally distinguished faculty including two Nobel Laureates in Physiology or Medicine. It is the founding developer of the Gleevec used in the treatment of chronic myeloid leukemia.

Mayo Clinic – Rochester of the Mayo Clinic Hospital in Rochester, MN, with over two thousand beds as a teaching and research hospital. It is composed of the Saint Marys Campus with its Mayo Eugenio Litta Children's Hospital as well as its Methodist campus forming an integral part of the Mayo Clinic's academic medical center. It is ranked first by the leading news reporting agency's Honor Roll as Best Hospitals in the United States.

Asan Medical Center is designated a tertiary teaching and research hospital of the University of Ulsan College of Medicine in Seoul, South Korea founded by Chung Ju-yung as part of the Asan Foundation. Inaugurated in 1989 under the original name of Seoul Central Hospital, it was later renamed in 2002 as the Asan Medical Center with a bed capacity of 2,700 and is the largest hospital in Korea. It holds a ranking of #5.

Institut Gustave Roussy is the first leader cancer-research hospital in Europe and holds a ranking among the top 3 best specialized hospitals in the world. It is a center for high quality patient care, research and teaching. It is known for the treatment of skin cancers such as melanoma, breast cancer, and lung cancer and it provides ready access to care with a distinguished internationally celebrated faculty. It is located in the Parisian area of France and is named for the acclaimed Swiss-French neuropathologist.

Charité – Universitätsmedizin Berlin is one of Europe's largest university hospitals, affiliated with Humboldt University and Free University Berlin. With numerous Collaborative Research Centers of the German Research Foundation it is one of Germany's most research-intensive medical institutions. From 2012 to 2022, it was ranked by *Focus* as the best of over 1000 hospitals in Germany. It has been ranked as the 5th best hospital in the world, and the best in Europe and it is located in Berlin.

Sidney Kimmel Comprehensive Cancer Center at Johns Hopkins University is an NCI-Designated Comprehensive Cancer Center in Baltimore, MD. It was established in 1973 and received its NCI designation that same year as one of the first designated cancer centers in the country. SKCCC is a member of the National Comprehensive Cancer Network, an alliance of 27 comprehensive cancer centers in the US. SKCCC is a prolific research institution. Many of the over 100 research laboratories are part of specialized research programs, including the Brain Cancer, Breast & Ovarian Cancer, Cancer Biology, Cancer Chemical & Structural Biology, Cancer Immunology, Cancer Molecular & Functional Imaging, Cancer Prevention & Control, Hematologic Malignancies & Bone Marrow Transplant, Prostate Cancer, and SPORE programs.

Princess Margaret Cancer Centre (previously, *Princess Margaret Hospital*) is a scientific research centre and a teaching hospital in Toronto, Ontario, Canada, affiliated with the University of Toronto Faculty of Medicine as part of the

University Health Network. The hospital now stands as the largest cancer centre in Canada and one of the five largest cancer centres in the world. Along with the Odette Cancer Centre, which is also associated with University of Toronto Faculty of Medicine and is independently the sixth largest cancer centre in North America, it forms one of the largest cluster of cancer hospitals in the world.

European Institute of Oncology (Italian: *Istituto Europeo di Oncologia*, IEO) is a non-profit private-law comprehensive cancer centre located in Milan, Italy. It is a clinic, a research centre and a training institution. IEO is a member of EU-LIFE, an alliance of leading life science research centres in Europe.[1] The European Institute of Oncology works on the prevention, diagnosis and treatment of cancer by developing clinical and scientific research coupled with organization and management. It provides a professional network for its members.

National Cancer Center Hospital (NCC) in Tokyo, Japan leads the nation's cancer treatment, prevention, control programs, research, and education Established by the Ministry of Health and Welfare in 1962. The leadership participates, and leads expert bodies appointed by the Ministry of Health, Labor and Welfare in the fight against cancer. Expertise is shared with the medical profession globally, with a focus on Asia. In 2010, it was designated an incorporated administrative agency (autonomous public service body), and then a national research and development agency in 2015, respectively remaining under the auspices of the Ministry of Health, Labor and Welfare.

Samsung Medical Center (SMC) is one of Korea's most renowned hospitals committed to excellence in providing the highest quality, compassionate care and service to patients. SMC was officially appointed as a medical evacuation hospital for the White House in 1996, in recognition of its medical expertise and dedication to a patient-centered culture. As nation's most comprehensive medical center, SMC offers variety of the latest diagnostic and treatment approaches through its Samsung Comprehensive Cancer Center, Proton Therapy Center and Heart Vascular and Stroke Institute, which are at the forefront of cancer treatment and heart & vascular diseases.

Royal Marsden Hospital is a specialist cancer treatment hospital in London adjacent to the Royal Brompton Hospital and is managed by the Royal Marsden NHS Foundation Trust. It was founded in 1851 as the Free Cancer Hospital and was the first hospital in the world dedicated to the study and treatment of cancer.

Cleveland Clinic Cancer Center, has more than 700 highly skilled doctors, researchers, nurses and technicians caring for thousands of patients each year. Cleveland Clinic Cancer Center unites clinicians and researchers in Taussig Cancer Institute and in Cleveland Clinic's 25 other clinical and surgical institutes, as well as cancer specialists at regional hospitals, health centers and at Cleveland Clinic Florida. The CCCC provides a range of services to patients including clinical trials and internationally-recognized cancer research efforts ensuring patients have access to the latest advances in cancer treatment, as well as a range of support programs helping patients navigate the challenges associated with a cancer diagnosis. Cleveland Clinic is recognized in the U.S. and throughout the world for its expertise and care.

Istituto Nazionale dei Tumori of Milan (INT) is the largest comprehensive cancer centre in Italy. Since its establishment, in 1928, this public institution has aimed to provide the highest standard of patient care while pursuing preclinical and clinical research and its swift translation into better prevention, diagnosis, therapy, rehabilitation, and quality of life. INT is an institute for scientific research, treatment and care, research at INT is funded by the National Ministry of Health and is supported by the regional authorities for its role in regional healthcare. Moreover, research is also substantially funded by numerous other bodies, both public -- such as the European Union and the Ministry of University and Research (MIUR) -- and private, in particular the Italian Association for Cancer Research (AIRC).

Peter MacCallum Cancer Centre, also known as the Peter MacCallum Cancer Institute and commonly abbreviated as Peter Mac, is an Australian oncology research institute, cancer treatment and professional oncologist training centre located in Melbourne, Victoria. The centre is named in honour of Sir Peter MacCallum. Since June 2016, the centre has been located within the Victorian Comprehensive Cancer Centre (VCCC) in Parkville. The centre is Australia's first public hospital dedicated to cancer treatment, research and education. Research programs at the centre include the Australian Cancer Research Foundation (ACRF) Cancer Cell Biology Program and the ACRF Victorian Centre for Functional Genomics in Cancer.

Roswell Park Comprehensive Cancer Center is a cancer research and treatment center located in Buffalo, New York. Founded by surgeon Roswell Park in 1898, the center was the first in the United States to specifically focus on cancer research. The center is usually called Roswell Park in short. The center, which conducts clinical research on cancer as well as the development new drugs, provides advanced treatment for all forms of adult and pediatric cancer, and serves as a member of the National Comprehensive Cancer Network. Roswell Park Comprehensive Cancer Center is as of 2019, the only upstate New York facility to hold the National Cancer Institute designation of "comprehensive cancer center".

Stanford University Medical Center is a medical complex which includes Stanford Health Care and Stanford Children's Health. It is consistently ranked as one of the best hospitals in the United States and serves as a teaching hospital for the Stanford University School of Medicine. In 2022-23, it was ranked 10th-best in the country.

Ruth and Raymond Perelman Center for Advanced Medicine is a specialized medical facility located at 34th Street and Civic Center Boulevard, on the former site of the Philadelphia Civic Center, on the campus of the Hospital of the University of Pennsylvania. The $302-million project was designed by Rafael Viñoly Architects and completed in 2008. It was the largest capital project ever undertaken by the University of Pennsylvania Health System, until the construction of The Pavilion. The center is home to Penn Medicine's Abramson Cancer Center, radiation oncology, cardiovascular medicine and an outpatient surgical pavilion. One of the most important parts of the Center for Advanced Medicine is the Roberts Proton Therapy Center which houses the largest proton therapy center associated with a medical center in the world. The proton therapy center will be used by both the Walter Reed Army

Medical Center and the Children's Hospital of Philadelphia, as well as the Penn Medicine to treat cancer patients.

University of Chicago Medicine Comprehensive Cancer Center is a collaborative cancer research center based in Hyde Park, Chicago, United States. The Comprehensive Cancer Center is affiliated with the University of Chicago. The Comprehensive Cancer Center was founded in 1973 as the University of Chicago Cancer Research Center, and, after earning its Comprehensive Cancer Center designation, was renamed the University of Chicago Medicine Comprehensive Cancer Center. The Comprehensive Cancer Center is one of 51 comprehensive cancer centers in the United States as designated by the National Cancer Institute of the National Institutes of Health. The first cancer research center director was John Ultmann whose specialty was the diagnosis, staging and treatment of Hodgkin's disease and non-Hodgkin's lymphoma, and the development of cancer chemotherapy.

UPMC Hillman Cancer Center, previously the University of Pittsburgh Cancer Institute (UPCI), is a National Cancer Institute (NCI)-designated Comprehensive Cancer Center located in the Hillman Cancer Center in the Shadyside neighborhood of Pittsburgh, adjacent to UPMC Shadyside. The only NCI-designated cancer center in Western Pennsylvania, Hillman is composed of collaborative academic and research efforts between the University of Pittsburgh, the University of Pittsburgh Medical Center (UPMC), and Carnegie Mellon University. Hillman provides clinical cancer care to some 74,000 patients treated at its facilities at both the Hillman Cancer Center location in the Shadyside neighborhood of Pittsburgh and at UPMC-affiliated sites throughout

Pennsylvania, New York, Ohio, and overseas locations. Founded in 1984, Hillman became the youngest cancer center in history to achieve NCI-designation. As of 2007, Hillman had received nearly $200 million in funding from the National Cancer Institute, which ranks it as one of the top ten cancer research institutes.

Vanderbilt-Ingram Cancer Center is an NCI-designated Comprehensive Cancer Center in Nashville, TN. It is part of the Vanderbilt University Medical Center. The Vanderbilt Cancer Center was established in 1993 and received its initial NCI designation in 1995. It was renamed the Vanderbilt-Ingram Cancer Center in 1999 after a significant donation from the Ingram family. The center received its NCI "comprehensive" cancer center status in 2001. VICC has more than 280 faculty members involved in the research and treatment of cancer. The center receives more than $140 million annually in federal research funding, landing it among the top ten in the nation for federal research grants.

Arthur G. James Cancer Hospital and Richard J. Solove Research Institute (commonly shortened to just The James) is part of The Ohio State University Wexner Medical Center and is one of the National Cancer Institute's Comprehensive Cancer Centers. It is named after Arthur G. James, the founder, who desired a cancer hospital in Columbus, Ohio, United States. The hospital treats cancer, and conducts research in the Solove Research Institute. The James receives donations through the Pelotonia biking event. In 2018, the James Cancer Hospital was designated a magnet hospital by the American Nurses Credentialing Center. With its expansion in 2014, it is now the third largest cancer hospital in the United States.

Alvin J. Siteman Cancer Center at Barnes-Jewish Hospital and Washington University School of Medicine is a cancer treatment, research and education institution with six locations in the St. Louis area. Siteman is the only cancer center in Missouri and within 240 miles of St. Louis to be designated a Comprehensive Cancer Center by the National Cancer Institute (NCI). Siteman is also the only area member of the National Comprehensive Cancer Network, a nonprofit alliance of 32 cancer centers dedicated to improving the quality and effectiveness of cancer care. In 2015 and 2020, Siteman received the highest rating possible - exceptional - by the NCI for cancer research. At Siteman's reviews leading to the ratings, researchers presented their findings in genomics, cancer imaging, cancer prevention and disparities, and the use of the body's immune system to fight cancer.

Koch Institute for Integrative Cancer Research at MIT is a cancer research center affiliated with the Massachusetts Institute of Technology (MIT) located in Cambridge, Massachusetts, United States. The institute is one of seven National Cancer Institute-designated basic laboratory cancer centers in the United States. The institute was launched in October 2007 with a $100 million grant from David H. Koch and the 180,000 square feet research facility opened in December 2010, replacing the MIT Center for Cancer Research (CCR).

St. Jude Children's Research Hospital is a pediatric treatment and research facility located in Memphis, Tennessee. Founded in 1962, it is a 501(c)(3) designated nonprofit medical corporation which focuses on children's catastrophic diseases, particularly leukemia and other cancers. In the 2021 fiscal year,

St. Jude received $2 billion in donations. Daily operating costs average $1.7 million, but patients are not charged for their care. St. Jude treats patients up to age 21, and for some conditions, up to age 25.

BIBLIOGRAPHY

Abuelo, C., Ashburner, J.M., Atlas, S.J., Knudsen, A., et al. (2020). "Colorectal Cancer Screening Patient Navigation for Patients with Mental Illness and/or Substance Use Disorder: Pilot Randomized Control Trial." *J Dual Diagn.* Oct; 16(4):438-446.

Ackerman, M.G., Shappiro, P.A., Coe, A., Trivedi, M.S., Crew, K.D. (2017). "The Impact of Mental Illness on Uptake of Genetic Counseling for Hereditary Breast Cancer and Ovarian Cancer in a Multiethnic Cohort of Breast Cancer Patients." *Breast J.* Sep; 23(5):519-524.

Ahlgren-Rimpilainen, A.J., Arffman, M., Suvisaari, J., Manderbacka, K., et al. (2020). "Excess Mortality from Breast Cancer in Female Breast Cancer Patients with Severe Mental Illness." *Psychiatry Res.* Aprl;286:112801.

Al-Qurayshi, Z., Rossi-Meyeer, M., Shama, M.A., Williams, A.M., et al. (2023). "Presentation and Outcomes of Otolaryngologic Surgeries in Patients with Mental Illness History." *Ann Otol Rhinol Laryngol.* Jun; 132(6):614-621.

Arffman, M., Manderbacka, K., Suvisaari, J., Koivunen, J., et al., (2019). "The impact of severe mental illness on lung cancer mortality of patients with lung cancer in Finland in

1990-2013: a register-based cohort study." *Eur J Cancer.* Sep;118:105-111.

Bentson, T.M., Floe, L.E., Bruun, J.M., Eriksen, J.G., Johnsen, S.P., et al. (2023). "Barriers in Cancer Trajectories of Patients with Pre-Existing Severe Mental Disorders: A Systematic Review." *Psychooncology.* Jun;32(6):862-874.

Bergamo C, Sigel K, Mhango G, Kale M, Wisnivesky JP. (2014). Inequalities in lung cancer care of elderly patients with schizophrenia: An observational cohort study. *Psychosom. Med.* 76: 215–220.

Bhattacharya, M., Parsons, H., Call, K., Blaes, A., McAlpine, D. et al. (2023). "Impact of a Pre-Existing Diagnosis of Mental Illness on Stage of Breast Cancer Diagnosis Among Older Women." *Breast Cancer Res Treat.* Jan;197(1):201-210.

Brutocao, C., Zaiem, F., Alsawas, M., Morrow, A.S., Murad, M.H., Javed, A. (2018). "Psychiatric Disorders in Women with Polycystic Ovary Syndrome." *Endocrine.* Nov. 62(2):318-325.

Caruso, Rosangela, Nanni, Mara G., Riba, Michelle B., Sabato, Silvana, Grassi, Luigi. (2017). "The Burden of Psychosocial Morbidity Related to Cancer: Patient and Family Issues." *Int Rev Psychiatry.* Oct; 29(5):389-402.

Cespedes, P., Sanchez-Martinez, V., Lera-Calatayud, G., Vila-Candel, R., et al. (2020). "Delay in the Diagnosis of Breast and Colorectal Cancer in People with Severe Mental Disorders." *Cancer Nurs.* Nov/Dec; 43(6):E356-E362.

Chang, C-K., Hayes, R.D., Broadbent, M.T.M., Hotopf, M., et al. (2014). "A Cohort Study on Mental Disorders Stage of Cancer at Diagnosis and Subsequent Survival." *BMJ Open.* Jan29;4(1):e04295.

Charlesworth, Laura, Fegan, Colette, Ashmore, Russell. (2023). "How Does Severe Mental Illness impact on Cancer Outcomes in Individuals with Severe Mental Illness and Cancer? A Scoping Review of the Literature." *J Med Imaging Radiat Sci.* June; 54(2S): S104-S114.

Chierzi, F., Stivanello, E., Musti, M.A., Perlangeli, V., Marzaroli, P., et al. (2023). "Cancer Mortality in Common Mental Disorders: A 10-Year Retrospective Cohort Study." *Soc Psychiatry Psychiatr Epidemiol.* Feb;58(2):309-318.

Chou, F.H-C., Tsai, K-Y., Wu, H-C., Shen, S-P. (2016). "Cancer in Patients with Schizophrenia; What is the Next Step?" *Psychiatry Clin Neurosci.* Nov;70(11):473-488.

Cui, Y., Lu, W., Shao, T., Zhuo, Z., Wang, Y., Zhang, W. (2023). "Severe Mental Illness and the Risk of Breast Cancer: A Two-Sample, two-Step Multivariable Mendelian Randomization Study." *PLoS One.* Sep 1; 18(9):e9291006.

Cunningham, R., Sarfati, D., Stanley, J., Peterson, D., Collings, S. (2015). "Cancer Survival in the Context of Mental Illness: A National Cohort Study." *Gen Hosp Psychiatry.* Nov-Dec; 37(6):501-506.

Davis, L.E., Bogner, E., Coburn, N.G., Hanna, T.P., Kurdyak, P., Groome, P.A., Mahar, A.L. (2020). "Stage at Diagnosis and

Survival in Patients with Cancer and a Pre-Existing Mental Illness: A Meta-Analysis." *J Epidemiol Community Health.* Jan; 74(1):84-94.

Deshpande, A.J., Bhandarkar, A., Bobo, W.V., Bydon, M., et al., (2023). "Examining the Relationship Between Severe Persistent Mental Illness and Surgical Outcomes in Women Undergoing Mastectomy for Breast Cancer." *Am J Surg.* Jul;226(1):4-10.

Etoh, T., Fujiwara, M., Yamada, Y., Wada, R., Higuchi, Y., et al. (2021). "Cancer Care for People with Mental Disorders: A Qualitative Survey Among Cancer Care and Psychiatric Care Professionals in Japan." *Psychooncology.* Dec;30(12):2060-2066.

Farland, D.C., Voigt, L., Alici, Y. (2021). "Decisional Capacity Determination and Serious Mental Illness in Oncology: Implications for Equitable and Beneficent Care." *Psychooncology.* Dec;30(12):2052-2059.

Feyera, F., Endeshaw, M., Kebede, Y., Tirfessa, K., Bekele, S.B. (2022). "The Magnitude of Common Mental Disorders and Associated Factors Among Cancer Patients at Black Lion Specialized Hospital, Addis Ababa, Ethiopia." *Cancer Control* Jan-Dec;29:1073274-8221127156.

Flores, E.J., Neil, J.M., Tiersma, K.M., Pappano, C.R., et al. (2021). "Feasibility and Acceptability of a Collaborative Lung Cancer Screening Educational Intervention Tailored for Individuals with Serious Mental Illness."

Flores, E.J., Park, E.R., Irwin, K.E. (2019). "Improving Lung Cancer Screening Access for Individuals with Serious Mental Illness." *J Am Coll Radiol.* Apr; 16(4 Pt B):596-600.

Forsythe LP, Kent EE, Weaver KE, et al. (2013). "Receipt of Psychosocial Care Among Cancer Survivors in the United States." *J Clin Oncol.* 31(16):1961-1969.

Fried, D.A., Sadeghi-Nejad, H., Gu, D., Zhou, S., He, W., Giordano, S.H. (2019). "Impact of Serious Mental Illness on the Treatment and Mortality of Older Patients with Locoregional high-grade (nonmetastatic) Prostate Cancer: Retrospective Cohort Analysis of 49,985 SEER-Medicare Patients Diagnosed Between 2006 and 2013." *Cancer Med.* May;8(5):2612-2622.

Fuller-Thomson, E., West, K.J. (2019). "Flourishing Despite a Cancer Diagnosis: Factors Associated with Complete Mental Health in a Nationally-Representative Sample of Cancer Patients aged 50 years and older." *Aging Ment Health.* Sep;23(9):1263-1274.

Geue, K., Brahler, E., Faller, H., Harter, M., Schulz, H., et al. (2018). Prevalence of Mental Disorders and Psychosocial Distress in German Adolescent and Young Adult Cancer Patients (AYA)." *Psychooncology.* July;27(7):;1802-1809.

Gillis, C., Ilie, G., Mason, R., Bailly, G., Lawren, J., et al. (2021). "Personality Traits and Urinary Symptoms Are Associated with Mental Health Distress in Patients with a

Diagnosis of Prostate Cancer." *Curr Oncol.* Aug 6; 28(4): 2993-3002.

Grassi, L., Caruso, R., Hammelef, K., Nanni, M.G., Riba, M. (2014). "Efficacy and safety of Pharmacotherapy in Cancer-Related Psychiatric Disorders Across the Trajectory of Cancer Care: A Review." *Int Rev Psychiatry.* Feb;26(1):44-62.

Grassi, L. (2020). "Psychiatric and Psychosocial Implications in Cancer Care: The Agenda of Psycho-Oncology." *Epidemiol. Psychiatr Sci.* Jan 9; 29:e89.

Grassi, Luigi and Riba, Michelle (2020). "Cancer and Severe Mental Illness: Bi-Directional Problems and Potential Solutions." *Psychooncology.* Oct; 29(10): 1445-1451.

Grassi, Luigi and Riba, Michelle (2021). "Disparities and Inequalities in Cancer Care and Outcomes in Patients with Severe Mental Illness: Call to Action." *Psychooncology.* Dec. 30(12): 1997-2001.

Grassi, L., Caruso, R., Biancosino, B., Murri, M.B., Riba, M., Meggiolaro, E., Ruffilli, F., Palagini, L., Nanni, M.G., Zayatta, S., Toffanin, T., Folesani, F., Zerbinati, L. (2021). "Knowledge About Rish Factors for Cancer and Cancer Risk Behavior Among Patients with Severe Mental Illness." *Psychooncology.* Dec; 30(12):2077-2081.

Grassi, Luigi, Folesani, Federica, Marella, Marco, Tiberto, Elisa, Riba, Michelle B., Bortolotti, Lisa, Toffanin, Tommaso, Palagini, Laura, Murri, Martino B., Biancosino, Bruno, Ferrar, Maria, Caruso, Rosangela. (2022). "Debating Euthanasia and

Physician-Assisted Death in People with Psychiatric Disorders." *R. Curr Psychiatry Rep.* June; 24(6): 325-335.

Grassi, L., Nanni, M.G., Caruso, R., Ounalli, H., Chochinov, H.M., Biancosino, B., Testoni, I., Murri, M.B., Bertelli, T., Palagini, L., De Padova, S., Tiberto, E. (2022). "A Comparison of Dignity Therapy Narratives Among People with Severe Mental Illness and People with Cancer." *Psychooncology.* Apri;32(4):676-679.

Gunther, M.P., Schulze, J.B., Kirchebner, J., Jordan, K.D., von Kanel, R., Euler, S. (2022). "Severe Mental Illness in Cancer is Associated with Disparities in Psycho-Oncological Support." *Current Problems in Cancer.* June; 46(3): 100849.

Gunther, M.P., Schulze, J.B., Jellestad, L. et al. (2021). "Mental Disorders, Length of Hospitalization, and Psychopharmacy: New Approaches to Identify Barriers to Psychological Support for Patients with Cancer." *Psychooncology.* Oct;30(10):1773-1781.

Happell, B., Scott, D., Platania-Phung, C. (2012). "Provision of Preventive Services for Cancer and Infectious Diseases among Individuals with Serious Mental Illness." *Arch Psychiat Nurs.* June; 26(3) 192-201.

Haskins, C.B., McDowell, B.D., Carnahan, R.M., Giedorowicz, J.G., et al. (2019). "Impact of Pre-existing Mental Illness on Breast Cancer Endocrine Therapy Adherence." *Breast Cancer Res Treat.* Feb;174(1):197-208.

Haskins, C.B., McDowell, B.D., Carnahan, R.M., Fiedorowicz, J.G., et al. (2021). "Breast Cancer Endocrine Therapy Adherence in Health Professional Shortage Areas: Unique Effects on Patients with Mental Illness." *J Psychosom Res.* Jan;140:110294.

Hemmington, A., Huang, D., Coomarasamy, C., Young, M.J., Consedine, N.S., Reynolds, L.M. (2020). "When Mental Illness and Cancer Collide: An Investigation of the Predictors of Outcomes for Cancer Patients with a History of Mental Health Problems." *Psychooncology.* Mar; 29(3):525-531.

Hicks, B.M., Busby, J., Mills, K., O'Neil, F.A., McIntosh, S.A., et al. (2020). "Post-Diagnostic Antipsychotic Use and Cancer Mortality: A Population Based Cohort Study." *BMC Cancer.* Aug 24;20(1):804.

Hu, Kejia, Wang, J., Sparen, P., Herweijer, E., Sjolander, A., et al. (2023). "Invasive Cervical Cancer, Precancerous leisons, and Cervical Screening Participation Among Women with Mental Illness in Sweden: A Population-Based Observational Study." *Lancet Public Health.* Apr;8(4):e-266-e275.

Hu, Siqi, Baraghoshi, D., Chang, C-P, Rowe, K., Snyder, J., et al. (2023). "Mental Health Disorders Among Ovarian Cancer Survivors in a Population-Based Cohort." *Cancer Med.* Jan;12(2):1801-1812.

Hyer, J.M., Kelly, E.P., Paredes, A.Z., Tsilmigras, D.I., Diaz, A., Pawlik, T.M. (2021). "Mental Illness is Associated with Increased Risk of Suicidal Ideation Among Cancer Surgical Patients." *A J Surg.* Jul; 222(1):126-132.

Iglay, K., Santorelli, M.L., Hirshfield, K.M., Williams, J.M., Rhoads, G.G., et al. (2017). "Diagnosis and Treatment Delays Among Elderly Breast Cancer Patients with Pre-Existing Mental Illness." *Breast Cancer Res Treat.* Nov; 166(1):267-275.

Iglay, K., Santorelli, M.L., Hirshfield, K.M., Williams, J.M., Rhoads, G.G., et al. (2017). "Impact of Preexisting Mental Illness on All-Cause and Breast Cancer-Specific Mortality in Elderly Patients with Breast Cancer." *J Clin Oncol.* Dec 20;35(36):4012-4018.

Irwin KE, Henderson DC, Knight HP, Pirl WF. (2014). "Cancer care for individuals with schizophrenia." *Cancer* 2014; 120: 323–334.

Irwin, K.E., Park, E.R., Fields, L.E., Corveleyn, A.E., Greer, J.A., Perez, G.K., Callaway, C.A., Jacobs, J.M., Nierenberg, A.A., Temel, J.S., Ryan, D.P., Pirl, W.F. (2019). "Bridge:Person-Centered Collaborative Care for Patients with Serious Mental Illness and Cancer." *Oncologist.* July; 24 (7): 901-910.

Irwin, K.E., Callaway, C.A., Corveleyn, A.E., Pappano, C.R., et al., 2022). "Study protocol for a randomized trial of bridge: Person-centered collaborative care for serious mental illness and cancer." *Contemp Clin Trials.* Dec;123:106975.

Ishikawa H, Yasunaga H, Matsui H, Fushimi K, Kawakami N. (2016). Differences in cancer stage, treatment and in-hospital mortality between patients with and without schizophrenia:

Retrospective matched-pair cohort study." *Br. J. Psychiatry* 208: 239–244.

James, M., Thomas, M., Frolov, L., Riano, N.S., Vittinghoff, E., et al. (2017). "Rates of Cervical Cancer Screening Among Women with Severe Mental Illness n the Public Health System." *Psychiatr Serv.* Aug 1;68(8):839-842.

Ji, X., Cummings, J.R., Marchak, J.G., Han, X., Mertens, A.C. (2020). "Mental Health Among Nonelderly Adult Cancer Survivors: A National Estimate." *Cancer.* Aug 15;126(16):3768-3776.

Jorgensen, Marie D., Mikkelsen, Ellen M., Erichen, Rune, Thomsen, Metta K. (2022). "Mental Illness and Participation in Colorectal Cancer Screening: A Scoping Review." *Scand J. Gastroenterol.* Oct: 57(10): 1216-1226.

Kahn, G.D., Tam, S.H., Felton, J.W., Westphal, J., Simon, G.E., et al. (2023). "Cancer and Psychiatric Diagnoses in the Year Preceding Suicide." *Cancer Med.* Feb;12(3):3601-3609.

Kaster, T.S., Sommer, J.L., Mota, N., Sareen, J., El-Gabalawy, R. (2019). "Post-Traumatic Stress and Cancer: Findings from a Cross-Sectional Nationally Representative Sample." *J Anxiety Disord.* Jun;65:11-18.

Kaul, S., Avila, J.C., Mutambudzi, M., Russell, H., Kirchhoff, A.C., Schwartz, C.L. (2017). "Mental Distress and Health Care Use Among Survivors of Adolescent and Young Adult Cancer: A Cross-Sectional Analysis of the National Health Interview Survey." Mar1:123(5):869-878.

Kerrison, R.S., Jones, A., Peng, J., Price, G., Verne, J., Barley, E.A., Lugton, C. (2023). "Inequalities in Cancer Screening Participation between Adults with and without Severe Mental Illness: Results from a Cross-Sectional Analysis of Primary Care Data on English Screening Programmes." *Br J Cancer.* Jul;129(1):81-93.

Keszte, J., Danker, H., Dietz, A., Meister, E., Pabst, F., et al. (2017). "Course of Psychiatric Comorbidity and Utilization of Mental Health Care After Laryngeal Cancer: A Prospective Cohort Study." *Eur Arch Otorhinolaryngol.* Mar;274(3):1591-1599.

Kim, H., Kim, K., Kim, Y.H. (2022). "Associations Between Mental Illness and Cancer: A Systematic Review and Meta-Analysis of Observational Studies." *Eur Rev Med Pharmacol Sci.* July; 26(14): 4997-5007.

Kirkoen, Benedicte, Berstad, Paula, Hoff, Geir, Bernkley, Tomm, Randel, Kristin R., Holme, Oyyind, de Lange, Thomas, Robb, Kathryn A., Botteri, Edoardo. (2023). "Type and Severity of Mental Illness and Participation in Colorectal Cancer Screening." *Am J Prev Med.* Jan; 64(1):76-85.

Kisely S, Forsyth S, Lawrence D. (2016). "Why do psychiatric patients have higher cancer mortality rates when cancer incidence is the same or lower?" *Aust. N. Z. J. Psychiatry* 50: 254–263.

Kisely, Steve, Alotiby, M.K.N., Protani, Melinda M., Soole, Rebecca, Arnautovska, Urska, Siskind, Dan. (2023). "Breast

Cancer Treatment Disparities in Patients with Severe Mental Illness: A Systematic Review and Meta-Analysis." *Psychooncology.* May; 32(5): 651-662.

Kittel, J.A., Seplaki, C.L., Van Wijngaarden, E., Richman, J., Magnuson, A., Conwell, Y. (2023). "Mental Health Outcomes and Correlates in Cancer Patients Entering Survivorship After Curative Treatment." *J Psychiatry Med.* Jul;58(4):325-338.

Kuhnt, S., Brahler, E., Faller, H., Harter, M., Keller, M., et al. (2016). "Twelve-Month and Lifetime Prevalence of Mental Disorders in Cancer Patients." *Psychother Psychosom.* 85(5):289-296.

Launders, Naomi, Scolamiero, Laura, Osborn, David P. J., Hayes, Joseph F. (2022). "Cancer Rates and Mortality in People with Severe Mental Illness: Further Evidence of Lack of Parity." *Schizophr Res.* Aug; 246: 260-267.

Lawrence, W.R., Kuliszewski, M.G., Hosler, A.S., Leinung, M.C., Zhang, X., et al. (2021). "Association Between Preexisting Mental Illnesses and Mortality Among Medicaid-Insured Women Diagnosed with Breast Cancer." *Soc Sci Med.* Feb;270:113643.

Leahy, D., Donnelly, A., Irwin, K., Alton, P.D. (2021). "Barriers and Facilitators to Accessing Cancer Care for People with Significant Mental Health Difficulties: A Qualitative Review and Narrative Systnesis." *Psychooncology.* Dec;30(12):2012-2022.

Lee, J.H., Ba, D., Liu, G., Leslie, D., Zacharia, B.E., Goyal, N. (2019). "Association of Head and Neck Cancer with Mental Health Disorders in a Large Insurance Claims Database." *JAMA Otolaryngol Head Neck Surg.* Apr 1;145(4):339-344.

Lee SA, Nam CM, Kim YH, Kim TH, Jan SI, Park EC. (2020). "Impact of onset of psychiatric disorders and psychiatric treatment on mortality among patients with cancer." *Oncologist.* 25(4):e733-e742.

Li, Z., Li, Y., Guo, L., Li, M., Yang, K. (2021). "Effectiveness of Acceptance and Commitment Therapy for Mental Illness in Cancer Patients: A Systematic Review and Meta-Analysis of Randomized Controlled Trials." *Int J Clin Pract.* Jun;75(6):e13982.

Lloyd, S., Baraghoshi, D., Tao, R., Garrido-Languna, I., et al. (2019). "Mental Health Disorders are More Common in Colorectal Cancer Survivors and Associated with Decreased Overall Survival." *Am J Clin Oncol.* Apr:42(4):355-362.

Lopes R, Soares R, Figueiredo-Braga M, Coelho R. (2014). "Schizophrenia and cancer: Is angiogenesis a missed link?" *Life Sci.* 97: 91–95.

Lu, D., Andersson, T.M.L., Fall, K., Hultman, C.M., Czen, K., Valdimarsdottir, U., Fang, F. (2016). "Clinical Diagnosis of Mental Disorders Immediately Before and After Cancer Diagnosis: A Nationwide Matched Cohort Study in Sweden." *JAMA Oncol.* Sep 1;29(9):1188-96.

Ma, K-J., Su, S-Y., Nie, D., Chung, W-S., Yao, C-Y., Wang, J-Y. (2023). "Disparities in the Medical Expenditures of Patients with Cancer and Concomitant Mental Disorder: Analyzing the Effects of Diagnosis Sequence Order." *BMC Health Serv Res.* Jan 27;23(1):92.

Mahar, A.L., Kurdyak, P., Hanna, T.P., Coburn, N.G., Groome, P.A. (2020). "The Effect of a evere Psychiatric Illness on Colorectal Cancer Treatment and Survival: A Population-Based Retrospective Cohort Study." *PLoS One.* Jul 29;15(7):e0235409.

Manderbacka, K., Arffman, M., Lumme, S., Suvisaari, J., et al. (2018). "The Effect of History of Severe Mental Illness on Mortality in Colorectal Cancer Cases: A Register-Based Cohort Study." *Acta Oncol.* Jun;57(6):759-764.

McFarland, D.C., Voigt, L., Alici, Y., 2021). "Decisional capacity determination and serious mental illness in oncology: Implications for equitable and beneficent care." Psychooncology. Dec;30(12):2052-2059.

McNally, Richard J. (2011). *What Is Mental Illness?* Cambridge, MA: Harvard University Press.

Millman, J., Galway, K., Santin, O., Reid, J. (2016). "Cancer and Serious Mental Illness-Patient, Caregiver and Professional Perspectives: Study Protocol." *J Adv Nurs.* Jan; 72(1):;217-26.

Mitchell, A.J., Santo Pereira, I.E., Yadegarfar, M., Pepereke, S., et al. (2014). "Breast Cancer Screening in Women with Mental

Illness: Comparative Meta-Analysis of Mammography Uptake." *Br J Psychiatry. Dec;205(6):428-435.*

Momen, N.C., Ernst, A., Arendt, L.H., Olsen, J., Li, J., et al. (2019). "Mental and Behavioural Disorders in the Children of Mothers Diagnosed with Cancer: A Danish Population-Based Register Study." *Psychooncology.* Feb;28(2):408-414.

Morgan, John H. (2019). *Clinical Psychotherapy: A History and Theory and Practice (from Sigmund Freud to Aaron Beck).* N. Fort Myers, FL: Wyndham Hall Press.

Morgan, John H. (2020). *The Scope of Modern Psychiatry: Treatment Options in Clinical Practice.* N. Fort Myers, FL: Wyndham Hall Press.

Morgan, John H. (2021). *The Damaged Self: Exploring the Psychopathology of a Diminished Life.* N. Fort Meyers, FL: Wyndham Hall Press.

Morgan, John H. (2022). *Schizophrenia: The Enduring Challenge to Psychiatric Practice.* N. Fort Myers, FL: Wyndham Hall Press.

Morgan, John H. (2023a). *Psychiatric Oncology: Critical Essays in the Psychosocial Spectrum of Cancer Care.* N. Fort Myers, FL: Wyndham Hall Press.

Morgan, John H. (2023b). *Cancer and Suicide: A Resource Compendium of Published Research.* N. Fort Myers, FL: Wyndham Hall Press.

Murphy, K.A., Stone, E.M., Presskreischer, R., McGinty, E.E., Daumit, L., Pollack, C.E. (2021). "Cancer Screening Among Adults With and Without Serious Mental Illness: A Mixed Methods Study." *Med Care.* April l; 59(4):327-333.

Murphy, K.A., Daumit, G.L., McGinty, E.E., Stone, E.M., Kennedy-Hendricks, A. (2021). "Predictors of Cancer Screening Among Black and White Maryland Medicaid Enrollees with Serious Mental Illness." *Psychooncology.* Dec; 30(12):2092-2098.

Murphy, Kerri A., Corveleyn, Amy E., Park, Elyse R., Irwin, Kelly E. (2023). "Challenges, Rewards, and Lessons Learned from Family and Community Caregivers of Individuals with Serious Mental Illness and Cancer." *Support Care Cancer.* Jul 26;31(8):492.

Ora Nakash, Itzhak Levav, Sergio Aguilar-Gaxiola, Jordi Alonso, et al., (2014). "Comorbidity of common mental disorders with cancer and their treatment gap: findings from the World Mental Health Surveys." *Psychooncology.* Jan;23(1):40-51.

Ng, H.S., Woodman, R., Koczwara, B. (2023). "Health Status and Mental Distress in People with Cancer and Comorbid Conditions: The Australian National Health Survey Analysis." *Cancer Med.* Aug;12(16):17225-17238.

O'Neill, S., Posada-Villa, J., Medina-Mora, M.E., Al-Hamzawi, A.O., et al. (2014). "Associations Between DSM-IV Mental Disorders and Subsequent Self-Reported Diagnosis of Cancer." *J Psychosom Res.,* Mar;76(3):207-212.

Paredes, A., Hyer, J.M., Tsilimigras, D.I., Palmer, E., Lustberg, M.B., Dillhoff, M.E., Cloyd, J.M., Tsung, Al., Ejaz, A., Gregorio, S W-D., Pawlik, T.M. (2021). "Association of Pre-Existing Mental Illness with All-Cause and Cancer-Specific mortality Among Medicare Beneficiaries with Pancreatic Cancer." *HPB (Oxford).* Mar; 23(3):451-458.

Park, S.J., Wai, A., Pavithran, K., Kunheri, B., Valsraj, K. (2021). "Cancer and Severe Mental Illness in Low- and Middle-income Countries: The Challenges and Outlook for the Future." *Psychooncology.* Dec; 30(12): 2002-2011.

Parpa, E., Tsilika, E., Gennimata, V., Mystakidou, K. (2015). "Elderly Cancer Patients' Psychopathology: A Systematic Review: Aging and Mental Health." *Arch Gerontol Geriatr.* Jan-Feb; 60(1):9-15.

Peterson, T. (2019). "Mental Illness Definition: What Is Mental Illness?" *HealthyPlace.* https://www.healthyplace.com/other-info/mental-illness-overview/mental-illness-definition-what-is-mental-illness.

Pham, H., Torres, H., Sharma, P. (2019). "Mental Health Implications in Bladder Cancer Patients: A Review." *Urol Oncol.* Feb; 37(2):97-107.

Protani, M.M., Alotiby, M.K.N., Seth, R., Lawrence, D., Jordan, S.J., Logan, H., Kendall, B.J., Siskind, D., Sara, G., Kisely, S. (2022). "Colorectal Cancer Treatment in People with Severe Mental Illness: A Systematic Review and Meta-Analysis." *Epidemiol Psychiat Sci.* Nov 17; 31:e82.

Protani, M.M., Jordan, S.J., Kendall, B.J., Siskind, D., et al. (2021). "Colorectal Cancer Outcomes in People with Severe Mental Illness Cohort (COSMIC): A Protocol for an Australian Retrospective Cohort Using Linked Administrative Data." *BMJ Open.* Jun 8;11(6):e044737.

Reavley NJ, Jorm AF. (2014). "The Australian public's beliefs about the causes of schizophrenia: associated factors and change over 16 years." *Psychiatry Res.*220: 609–614.

Ross, E., Maguire, A., Mairs, A., Hall, C., Donnelly, M.J.C., O'Reilly, D.P.J. (2021). "Disparities in Breast Cancer Screening Uptake for Women with Mental Illness in the United Kingdom." *Am J Prev Med.* Mar;60(3):e123-e130.

Salm, S., Blaschke, K., Ihle, P., Schubert, I., Dresen, A., et al. (2021). "Mental Disorders and Utilization of Mental Health Services in Newly Diagnosed Cancer Patients: An Analysis of German Health Insurance Claims Data." *Psychooncology.* Mar;30(3):312-320.

Sathianathen, N., Fan, Yunhua, Jarosek, S.L., Konety, Isha, Weight, Christopher J., Vinogradov, Sophia, Konety, Badrinath R. (2020). "Disparities in Bladder Cancer Treatment and Survival Amongst Elderly Patients with a Pre-Existing Mental Illness." *Eur Urol Focus.* Nov 15;6(6): 1180-1187.

Saxena, P.U.P., Kulharni, V., Thapar, R., Pai, K., Gupta, A., Kotian, H. (2018). "Assessment of Spectrum of Mental Disorders in Cancer Patients." Oct-Dec;14(6):1312-1315.

Schomerus G, Angermeyer MC, Baumeister SE, Stolzenburg S, Link BG, Phelan JC. (2016). "An online intervention using information on the mental health-mental illness continuum to reduce stigma." *Eur. Psychiatry*. 32: 21–27.

Shinden, Y., Kijima, Y., Hirata, M., Nakajo, A., Tanoue, K., et al. (2017). "Clinical Characteristics of Breast Cancer Patients with Mental Disorders." *Breast.* Dec;36:39-43.

Shirama, F.H., Silva, T.B., Dos Santos, J.C., de Oliveira, P.A., et al. (2019). "Factors Associated with Common Mental Disorders and Use of Psychiatric Drugs in Cancer Outpatients." *Arch Psychiatr Nurs.* Oct;33(5):88-93.

Siantz, E., Wu, B., Shiroiski, M., Vora, H., Idos, G. (2017). "Mental Illness is Not Associated with Adherence to Colorectal Cancer Screening: Results from the California Health Interview Survey." *Dig Dis Sci.* Jan;62(1):224-234.

Solmi, M., Firth, J., Miola, A., Fornaro, M., Frison, E., et al. (2020). "Disparities in Cancer Screening in People with Mental Illness across the World versus the General Population: Prevalence and Comparative Meta-Analysis Including 4,717,839 People." *Lancet Psychiatry.* Jan;7(1):52-63.

Stedman, Thomas Lathrop (2005, 2nd ed.) *The American Heritage Stedman's Medical Dictionary.* Boston, MA: Houghton Mifflin.

Steffens, E.B., Park, E.R., Muzikanshy, A., Streck, J.M. et al. (2023). "Patients with Serious Mental Illness Can Engage in Tobacco Treatment Trials and Tobacco Cessation Interventions

During Cancer Treatment." *JCO Oncol Pract.* Feb;19(2)e238-3-247.

Sykes, K., Tuschick, E., Giles, E., Kanmodi, K.K., Barler, J. (2022). "A Protocol to Identify the Barriers and Facilitators for People with Severe Mental Illness and/or Learning Disabilities for Person Centred Cancer Screening Services (PECCS)." *PLoS One.* Nov. 30; 17(11):eo278238.

Tamauchi, S., Kajiyama, H., Moriyama, Y., Yoshihara, M., et al. (2019). "Relationship Between Preexisting Mental Disorders and Prognosis of Gynecologic Cancers: A Case-Control Study." *J Obstet Gynaecol Res.* Oct;45(10):2082-2087.

Thomsen, M.K., Jorgensen, M.D., Pedersen, L., Erichsen, R., et al. (2023). "Mental Disorders, Participation, and Trajectories in the Danis Colorectal Cancer Programme: A Population-Based Cohort Study." *Lancet Psychiatry.* Jul;10(7):518-527.

Toender, A., Munk-Olsen, T., Vestergaard, M., Larsen, J.T., et al. (2018). "Impact of Severe Mental Illness on Cancer Stage at Diagnosis and Subsequent Mortality: A Population-Based Register Study." *Schizophr Res.* Nov;201:62-69.

Tuesley, K.M., Jordan, S.J., Siskind, D.J., Kendall, B.J., Kisely, S. (2019). "Colorectal, Cervical and Prostate Cancer Screening in Australians with Severe Mental Illness: Retrospective Nation-Wide Cohort Study." *Aust N Z J Psychiatry.* Jun; 53(6)550-558.

Vancampfort D, Rosenbaum S, Probst M *et al.* Promotion of cardiorespiratory fitness in schizophrenia: A clinical overview and meta-analysis. *Acta Psychiatr. Scand.* 2015; 132: 131–143.

Van Warmerdam, J., Sutradhar, R., Kurdyak, P., Lau, C., Pole, J.D., et al. (2020). "Long-Term Mental Health Outcomes in Mothers and Siblings of Children with Cancer: A Population-Based, Matched Cohort Study." *J Clin Oncol.* Jan 1;38(1):51-62.

Vehling, S., Mehnert-Theuekauf, A., Glaesmer, H., Bokemeyer, C., et al. (2021). "Thoughts of Death and Suicidality Among Patients with Cancer: Examining Subtypes and Their Association with Mental Disorders." *Psychooncology.* Dec;30(12):2023-2031.

Walker, Z.J., Xue, S., Jones, M.P., Ravindran, A.V. (2021). "Depression, Anxiety, and Other Mental Disorders in Patients with Cancer in Low- and Lower-Middle-Income Countries: A Systematic Review and Mta-Analysis. *JCO Glob Oncol.* Jul;7:123;3-1250.

Weinstein, L.C., Stefancic, A., Cunningham, A.T., Hurley, K.E., Cabassa, L.J., Wender, R.C. (2016). "Cancer Screening, Prevention, and Treatment in People with Mental Illness." *CA Cancer J Clin.* Mar-Apr;66(2):134-151.

Woodhead, C., Cunningham, R., Ashworth, M., Barley, E., Stewart, R.J., Henderson, M.J. (2016). "Cervical and Breast Cancer Screening Uptake Among Women with Serious Mental

Illness: A Data Linkage Study. *BMC Cancer.* Oct 21;16(1):819.

Wu CS, Gau SS. (2016). "Association between antipsychotic treatment and advanced diabetes complications among schizophrenia patients with type 2 diabetes mellitus." *Schizophr. Bull.* 42: 703–711.

Yamada, Y., Fujiwara, M., Etoh, T., Wada, R., Inoue, S., et al. (2022). "Issues of Cancer Care in People with Mental Disorders as Perceived by Cancer Care Providers: A Quantitative Questionnaire Survey." *Psychooncology.* Sep;31(9):1572-1580.

Yamada, Y., Fujiwara, M., Etoh, T., Wada, R., Inoue, S., et al. (2023). "Perceptions Towards Issues in Cancer Care for People with Mental Illness Among Psychiatric Care Providers: A Questionnaire Study. *Psychooncology.* July;32(7):1022-1029.

Yarborough, B.J.H., Hanson, G.C., Perrin, N.A., Stumbo, S.P., Green, C.A. (2018). "Colorectal Cancer Screening Completion Among Individuals With and Without Mental Illnesses: A Comparison of 2 Screening Methods." *Am J Health Promot.* May;32(4):925-93l.

Zhu, J., Fang, F., Sjolander, A., Fall, K., Adami, H.O., Valdimarsdottir, V. (2017). "First-Onset Mental Disorders After Cancer Diagnosis and Cancer-Specific Mortality: A Nationwide Cohort Study." *Ann Oncol.* Aug 1;28(8):1964-1969.

Zhu, J., Sjolander, A., Fall, K., Valdimarsdottir, U., Fang, F. (2018). "Mental Disorders Around Cancer Diagnosis and Increased Hospital Admission Rate – A Nationwide Cohort Study of Swedish Cancer Patients." *BMC Cancer.* Mar 27;18(1):322.

INDEX

ABOUT THE AUTHOR

John Henry Morgan, Ph.D.(Hartford), D.Sc.(London), Psy.D.(FH/Oxford), Senior Fellow in Behavioral Science *emeritus,* Foundation House/Oxford (UK), is a clinical psychopathologist specializing in psychiatric oncology and personality disorders. He was educated at Harvard, Yale, and Princeton in the behavioral sciences from which he held six postdoctoral research appointments. Dr. Morgan recently retired from teaching a doctoral-level seminar for 20 years in the International Summer Program of Oxford University (1995-2015) during which time he also served concurrently as a Postdoctoral Visiting Scholar at New York University (2010) as well as holding three appointments as Postdoctoral Research Scholar at the University of Chicago (1976;1986; 1992). Prior to his years of teaching at Oxford University (1995-2015), he held an appointment as the National Science Foundation Science Faculty Fellow at the University of Notre Dame (1980) and held three successive postdoctoral appointments as Visiting Scholar to Harvard University (1998; 2011; 2015). Most recently, Dr. Morgan has been named to the Board of Editors of the *International Journal of Psychiatry in Medicine,* a leading medical journal published by Sage Publications.

RELATED BOOKS BY THE AUTHOR

(published by Wyndham Hall Press, available at Amazon Books)

- *Cancer and Suicide: A Resource Compendium of Published Research*
- *Psychiatric Oncology: Critical Essays in the Psychosocial Spectrum of Cancer Care*
- *Schizophrenia: The Enduring Challenge to Psychiatric Practice*
- *A Summary Guide to the Collected Works of Sigmund Freud*
- *Sigmund Freud Comprehensive Reference Dictionary of Psychoanalysis*
- *Harry Stack Sullivan Encyclopedic Dictionary of Interpersonal Psychotherapy*
- *Psychopathology: A Clinical Guide to Personality Disorders*
- *Clinical Psychotherapy: A History of Theory and Practice*
- *Understanding Ourselves: Essays in the History & Philosophy of the Social Sciences*
- *Child Psychopathology in Clinical Practice: The Psychoanalytic Theories of Karen Horney, Melanie Klein, and Anna Freud*
- *The Learning Spectrum in Child Development: Developmental Psychology in Maria Montessori, Jean Piaget, and Erik Erikson*

- *Geriatric Psychotherapy: Essays in Clinical Practice and Counseling Psychology*
- *The Scope of Modern Psychiatry: Treatment Options in Clinical Practice*
- *The Damaged Self: Exploring the Psychopathology of a Diminished Life*
- *The Morgan Reader: A Compendium of Scholarly Papers*

Made in United States
Orlando, FL
04 November 2026

90202246R10192